GOLD'S GYM
NUTRITION BIBLE

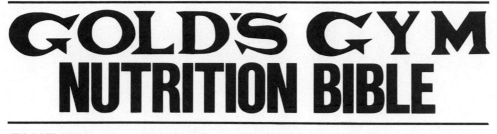

GOLD'S GYM
NUTRITION BIBLE

TIM KIMBER, BILL REYNOLDS, PETER GRYMKOWSKI, AND ED CONNORS

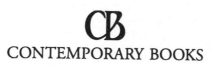

CONTEMPORARY BOOKS

Library of Congress Cataloging-in-Publication Data

Gold's Gym nutrition bible.

    Bibliography: p.
      1. Bodybuilders—Nutrition.   I. Kimber, Tim.
TX361.B46G65   1986   641.3'024796   86-16604
ISBN 0-8092-5188-4 (pbk.)

35   34   33   32   31   30   29   28   27   26   25   24   23   22   21   20   19   18

CONTENTS

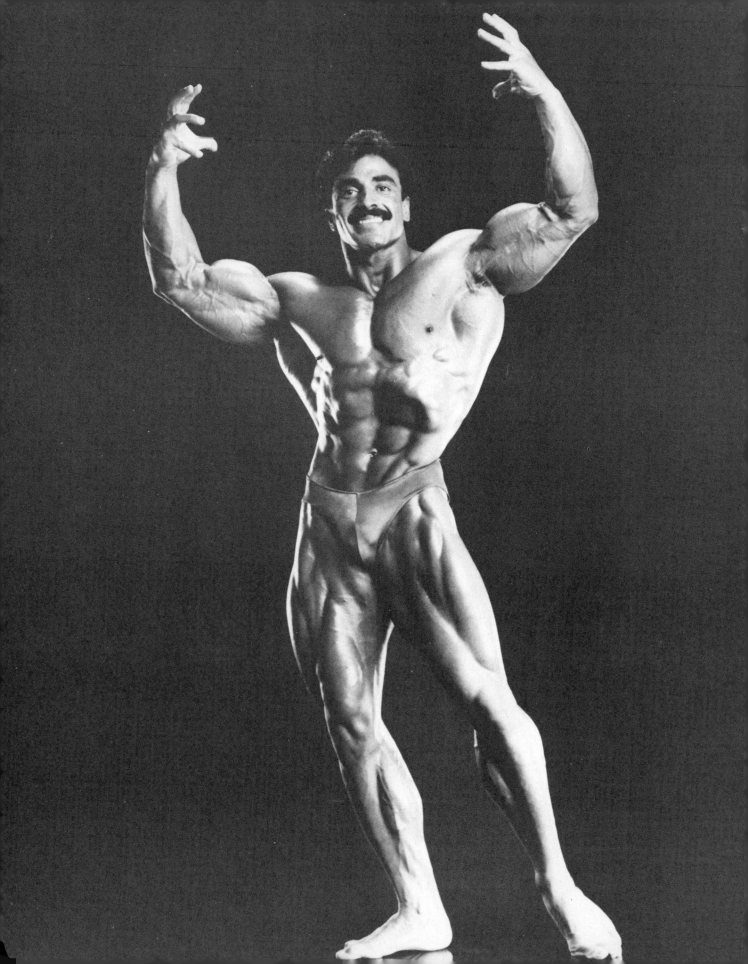

1
INTRODUCTION TO BODYBUILDING NUTRITION

You truly are what you eat, and bodybuilding nutrition is between 50 percent and 80 percent a function of the diets you follow. To give you an overview of how important proper nutrition is to a serious bodybuilder, we could ask no greater experts than a Mr. Olympia and a Ms. Olympia for the lowdown.

"Nutrition is at least 50 percent of the battle during my off-season cycle," reveals Lee Haney (American and World Heavyweight Champion and twice Mr. Olympia). "And as a competition approaches, diet becomes increasingly important to me, until it is up to 80 percent of the battle. Through extensive experimentation, I have discovered that I can train as hard as a Trojan in the gym and have a perfect mental attitude, but everything will go for nothing if my diet is faulty. Proper nutrition is the key to bodybuilding success at every level of competition, from local novice shows right up to the Mr. Olympia competition every year."

"The gym isn't the only place where you build your muscles," concurs Corinna Everson (National Champion and twice Ms. Olympia). "That happens in your kitchen too, but only if yours is stocked with the right foods and supplements necessary to build stamina, strength, and muscle tissue. The correct combination of proteins, carbohydrates, fats, water, vitamins, minerals, and enzymes is vitally important in the overall training philosophy of all successful bodybuilders. I know I would never have won my Ms. Olympia titles if I ate doughnuts and hamburgers and drank soft drinks!"

Everything you eat affects your body, so you might as well eat good bodybuilding foods. As former Mr. California and Mr. America, Dale Adrian, said, "I eat for function, not for taste. My body requires only pure foods with the potential of building greater muscle mass and quality. What appeals to me is wholesome protein foods, complex and simple carbohydrates, a minimum of animal fats, at least 12 glasses of pure water per day, fresh vegetables and fruit, crisp salads, nuts, seeds, grains, vitamins, minerals, and enzymes. These are the foods that build bodies, so stick with them if you genuinely desire to develop a championship physique."

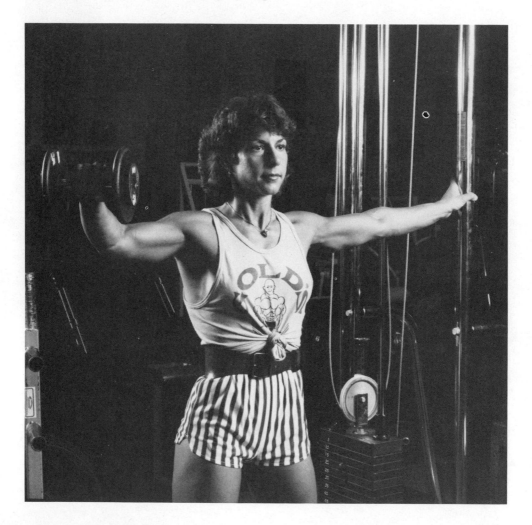

The information presented in this book will give you terrific impetus to succeed as a bodybuilder. But it won't work for you if you insist on eating junk foods every day, or even only one or two days per week. Follow our nutritional advice for bodybuilders, however, and you will become a champion much more quickly than those errant men and women who refuse to maintain a healthy, muscle-building diet.

We have covered a wide range of bodybuilding nutrition topics in this book, including such nutrients as protein, fats, carbohydrates, fiber, water, vitamins, minerals, and enzymes. Other topics discussed in this book include instinctive diet and supplementation, diet and exercise for weight gain, diet and exercise for fat loss, precontest diet, how to eat out safely, carbohydrate loading, how to manipulate your body's water balance, cycle dieting, how to improve energy levels, food allergies, vegetarian bodybuilding, detoxifying your body, and the mental side of bodybuilding nutrition. The book concludes with a collection of 17 recipes contributed by top bodybuilders who either currently train at Gold's Gym or have trained at Gold's in the past.

You should first read this book in its entirety to gain an overview of bodybuilding nutrition. Then you can go back and study each chapter in detail in order to master those topics that are most vital to your bodybuilding efforts. Finally, you can continue your study of bodybuilding nutrition by reading the diet articles published in *Muscle & Fitness* magazine and *Flex* magazine, plus some of the many other books published on bodybuilding nutrition.

You won't become a nutrition expert overnight, but all of the study time you spend learning about bodybuilding nutrition will be a great investment in your future as a competitor in our sport. After all, nutrition is at least 50% of the battle in becoming a top bodybuilder. Let's go for it the Gold's Gym way!

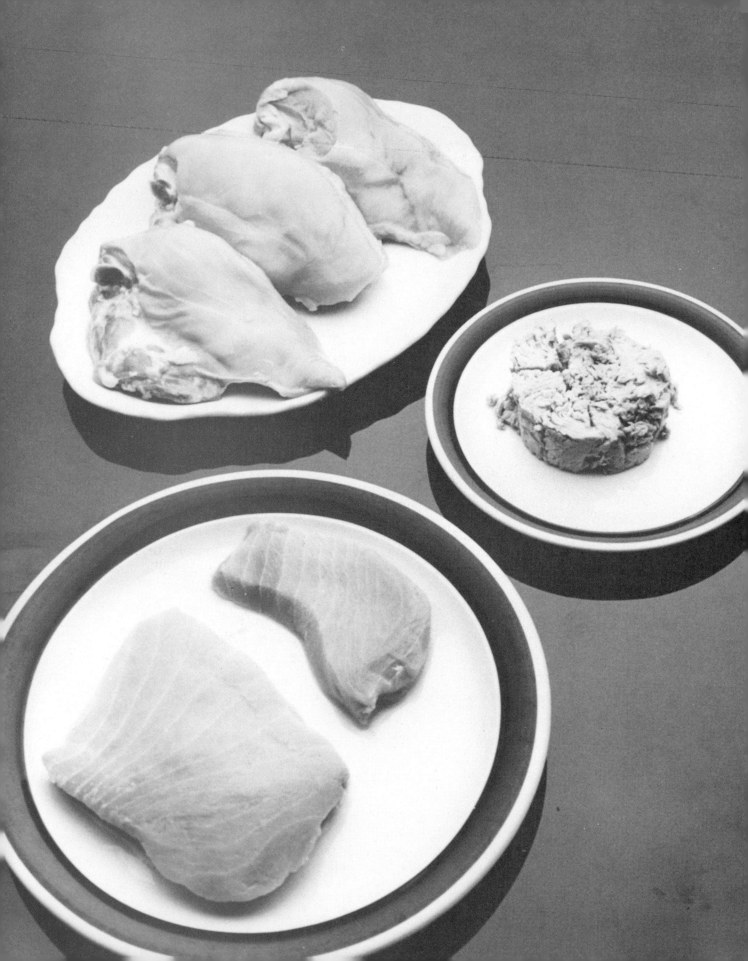

2
PROTEIN

A champion bodybuilder pays more attention to the protein in his or her diet than to any other nutrient because protein is the primary nonwater constituent of skeletal muscles. In their quest for bigger and more defined muscles, bodybuilders around the world have made millionaires of distributors of protein supplements, unwittingly paying for powders and pills that do little more than exhaust bank accounts.

The United States Food and Drug Administration (FDA) has established an Adult Minimum Daily Requirement (AMDR) for protein of one gram per kilogram of body weight (one kilogram equals 2.2 pounds), or slightly more than 0.45 grams per pound of body weight. While promoters of protein supplements will tell you that a bodybuilder needs three to five times the AMDR for protein in order to make acceptable gains, there is no hard experimental evidence to indicate that bodybuilders in heavy training need anything more than the AMDR for protein.

Even an average person consumes about two times as much protein each day as he or she needs. And bodybuilders eat more protein each day than do normal people. But excess protein can be turned into body fat just like excess fat can. When a bodybuilder consumes a diet that is excessively high in both proteins and fats, he or she will find it very difficult to achieve a hard and muscular appearance to go with the high degree of muscle mass he or she has achieved.

A diet excessively high in protein will also place a strain on the liver and kidneys, a fact you should take into consideration when choosing the foods you plan to eat, plus the type and amount of protein supplement you plan to take. An excessive intake of low-quality food, then, will be a health risk rather than a positive factor in your overall dietary philosophy.

Unlike some nutrients, protein cannot be stored in your body. It must be consumed in adequate supplies throughout the day in order to provide the tissue-building needs your workouts have stimulated. And, the protein you consume must be of high biological quality so that a maximum amount of it is used each time you eat.

Protein consists of 22 basic building blocks called amino acids. Nine amino acids cannot be manufactured within your body, and therefore must be consumed in food throughout the day. These nine are called essential amino acids. The other 13 aminos—called nonessential amino acids—can be manufactured within your body from the foods you consume in the course of a day.

The 22 amino acids can be combined in a large number of configurations—over 1,600—within your body. When those proteins containing all of the essential amino acids are nearly in the same conformation as the proteins in your body's tissues, the protein food has high biological quality.

This brings us to the concept of Protein Efficiency Ratio (PER). The PER scale was established as a means of evaluating the relative digestability and assimilability of a wide variety of protein foods. Egg white is at the top end of the PER scale, and it has been assigned a value of 1.0. Egg white is followed in descending order by fish meal and caseine, the protein found in milk.

In terms of PER, animal-source proteins are at the high end of the scale, while vegetable-source proteins lie at the low end. And white meats generally have higher PER ratings than red meats. You will find this information valuable when planning your meals.

When you choose a protein supplement, the best quality of protein will be egg white powder. But egg white powder is highly expensive and is in small supply even in so-called milk and egg protein powders. Normally the milk and egg protein powders sold in health food stores are about 97% to 99% caseine. But milk and egg protein powders are usually your best buy when seeking a protein supplement.

Protein powders made up from such vegetable-source foods as soybeans, yeast, and sesame seeds are of lower biological quality than milk and egg protein powders. But if you happen to be a vegetarian who doesn't consume milk or eggs, you will want to pick a protein powder made from soybeans, yeast, and/or sesame seeds.

Amino acid capsules can vary widely in PER as a function of the combination and amounts of various individual aminos. We will talk about amino acid supplements in some detail later in this chapter.

PROTEIN AND FATS

If you wanted to avoid food supplements, the best sources of dietary protein would be egg whites, fish, and broiled chicken or turkey breast meat that has been cooked with the skin

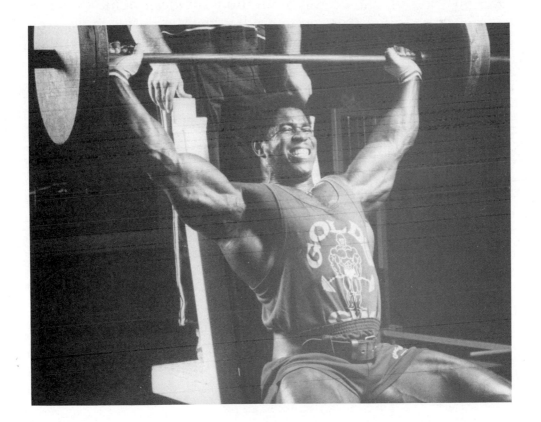

removed first. These are the best dietary protein foods in terms of both biological quality and low fat content.

A big problem with many of the protein foods in a body-builder's diet is that these foods are too high in fat content to suit a serious athlete's nutritional needs. So you need to be picky when deciding which foods to include in your daily diet.

Egg whites are almost pure protein of superior biological quality. And egg whites have no fats in them, so the calories you consume are virtually all protein. You can rely on egg whites for your dietary protein needs during both off-season mass-building and precontest defining cycles.

Fish is high in protein and also relatively low in fats, so you can also rely on fish protein during both off-season and precontest dietary cycles. By looking through caloric tables, you can find which fish dishes have the lowest fat content. Fish protein is very good for bodybuilders, but the protein in other seafood (shellfish, crustaceans) is of slightly lesser biological quality.

Poultry that has been cooked without the fatty skin is somewhat higher in fat calories than is fish, but it is still the protein food of choice for many bodybuilders peaking for a competition. In general, white poultry meat is somewhat lower in calories than dark meat, although fatty poultry like duck and goose can have white meat that is higher in caloric content than the dark meat of chicken.

Dairy foods can also be good sources of dietary protein in a bodybuilder's diet when steps have been taken to limit their fat content. Fat can be extracted from milk and set aside for the production of butter. The resulting foods that are made from nonfat milk have a high protein content in relation to calories.

Vegetarian foods have very little fat content, but they also don't contain much protein. And the protein you do find in vegetable foods is of relatively low biological quality. So you will need to consume vegetarian protein foods in combination with animal proteins to complete the vegetarian protein's amino acid balance by adding essential amino acids. Or, you will need to consume vegetarian foods in combination with other vegetarian-source proteins to help complete the protein combinations of each vegetarian protein being combined.

The best animal-vegetable protein combinations are as follows:

Milk + rice
     + legumes (kidney beans, navy beans, lima beans,
          pinto beans, soybeans, peanuts)
     + wheat

Eggs + rice
     + legumes
     + wheat

Meat + rice
     + legumes
     + wheat

When you combine vegetable-source proteins, you will obtain the most complete dietary protein with these combinations:

Rice + legumes
     + sesame seeds
     + wheat & soybeans

Wheat + rice & soybeans
     + peanuts & soybeans
     + legumes
     + soybeans & sesame seeds

Legumes + rice
     + corn
     + wheat
     + sesame seeds
     + oats
     + barley

We recommend an eclectic diet, one that includes all possible nutrients. So if you weight your diet heavily in animal proteins

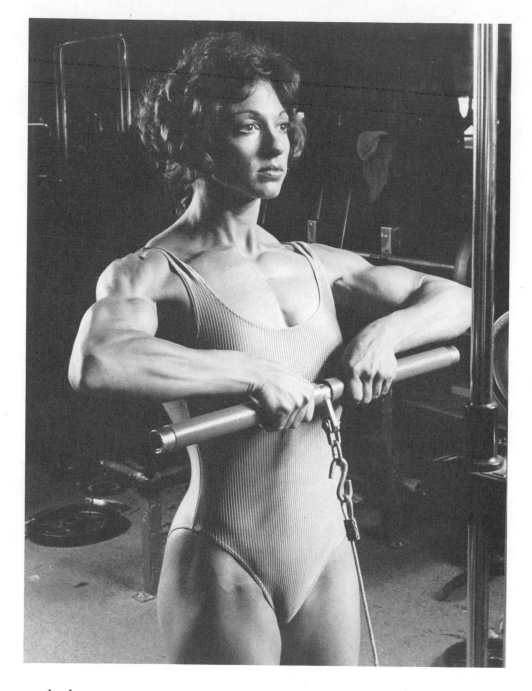

and also consume some vegetarian-source proteins with the animal proteins, your diet will have sufficient high-quality protein for muscle building.

AMINO ACID SUPPLEMENTS

Free-form amino acids—available in either powder or capsules—are one of the newest and best food supplements. A correct mix of high-grade individual aminos needs no digestion and passes directly into the bloodstream to provide a hard-training bodybuilder with aminos for tissue repair and muscle hypertrophy. Indeed, amino acids of pharmaceutical grade can be held under your tongue and passed directly through the membranes of your mouth and into your bloodstream, bypassing the digestive tract.

There are a lot of ripoffs in amino acid sales, primarily in the grades and formulas for amino acid mixes. There are three grades of amino acids available to food supplement distributors: food grade, pharmaceutical grade, and pharmaceutical I.V. grade. Most amino acid formulas—even those that are highly priced and whose promoters trumpet their high value to bodybuilders—are made from food grade amino acids, the cheapest type of aminos available. Only a few use pharmaceutical grade amino acids, since they are costly.

You can tell whether the amino acid supplement you might wish to purchase is an inferior formulation from the absence of such expensive individual aminos as lysine, tryptophan, arginine, ornithine, phenylalanine, and tyrosine. If the formulation lacks these aminos—or has very low milligram values in comparison to the other amino acids included in the formula—you should think twice about purchasing it.

We also suggest that you avoid predigested amino acids, which have relatively low assimilability and lack any amount of natural tryptophan. These amino acids are manufactured either by bathing cattle by-products (hides, hooves, lips, and a lot of other unmentionable components) in acid and later drawing off the resulting aminos, or by enzymatic breakdown techniques. Predigested aminos are sold in health food stores and are used as a foul-tasting drink by the spoonful or gulpful. We don't recommend them to anyone.

In contrast, free form aminos are L-configuration amino acids manufactured in Japan using a process called biological fermentation. In literature provided by Integrated Health, Inc., this process is described: "Microorganisms are introduced into a certain nutrient medium (e.g., sugar beets, molasses, etc.). This medium serves as their food for growth and reproduction. The end product of biological fermentation is the biologically active L-form amino acids. By ingesting amino acids in their singular free forms, body energy is conserved through the alleviation of further digestion."

When food supplement companies don't advertise and still gain large numbers of customers who are top bodybuilders, they sell amino acid capsules that do the job. One such company is Integrated Health, Inc., 1661 Lincoln Blvd., Santa Monica, CA 90404. (Marjorie Tyson, president, will be happy to send you literature on their aminos and other food products.) Integrated Health food products are also available at many Gold's Gym outlets around the United States and Canada.

"Our amino acid formulations are relatively expensive," Marjorie Tyson told us, "because they are of pharmaceutical grade. We sell aminos to the medical community, so we can't afford a goof. Lesser grades of amino acids often contain contaminants. With the grade we use, there is a uniformity of crystalline structure and no contaminants. They are guaranteed pyrosine free.

"Our amino acid products are manufactured using no heat, pressure, binders, preservatives, sugar, or coloring agents. The amino acids also do not come from soy, wheat, milk, meat, vegetables, yeast, or corn, so they are useful for vegetarians and individuals sensitive to the previously mentioned foods."

In working with scores of top bodybuilders (e.g., Frank Zane, Mike and Ray Mentzer, Andreas Cahling, Chris Glass, and many others) Ms. Tyson has determined that bodybuilders particularly need L-tryptophan, L-phenylalanine, L-tyrosine and para-aminobenzoic acid (PABA). She also suggests consuming amino acids with a dilute carbohydrate fluid (four ounces of apple, cranberry, or grape juice diluted with four ounces of pure water) to provide an internal source of calories, which facilitates absorption and assimilation.

When you are carb loading, amino acids provide an excellent complement to the complex carbs you consume, thereby sparing your muscle tissue from being catabolized to supply your energy needs. Simply consume complex carbs (e.g., rice, potatoes) with two to three high-grade amino acid capsules for each of five to eight small meals the day before your competition.

"When you begin using quality amino acids," Marjorie Tyson asserts, "you will notice a difference in your energy, muscle quality, and sense of well-being in only two or three days. And these will be more significant if your body is deficient in various aminos and other nutrients. We give a blood test which can pinpoint deficiencies in certain amino acids. We test for 44 values, including all 22 amino acids and intermediates like muscle tissue metabolites and ammonia. And once deficiencies have been identified, specific individual amino acids can be taken to erase the deficiencies."

In practical application, good quality amino acid capsules will provide bodybuilders with a variety of benefits, including higher workout energy, a better pump from workouts, more mental alertness, fewer hunger pangs when dieting, and bigger, better quality muscles. These wide-ranging benefits have been confirmed in actual practice by a variety of Gold's Gym champions.

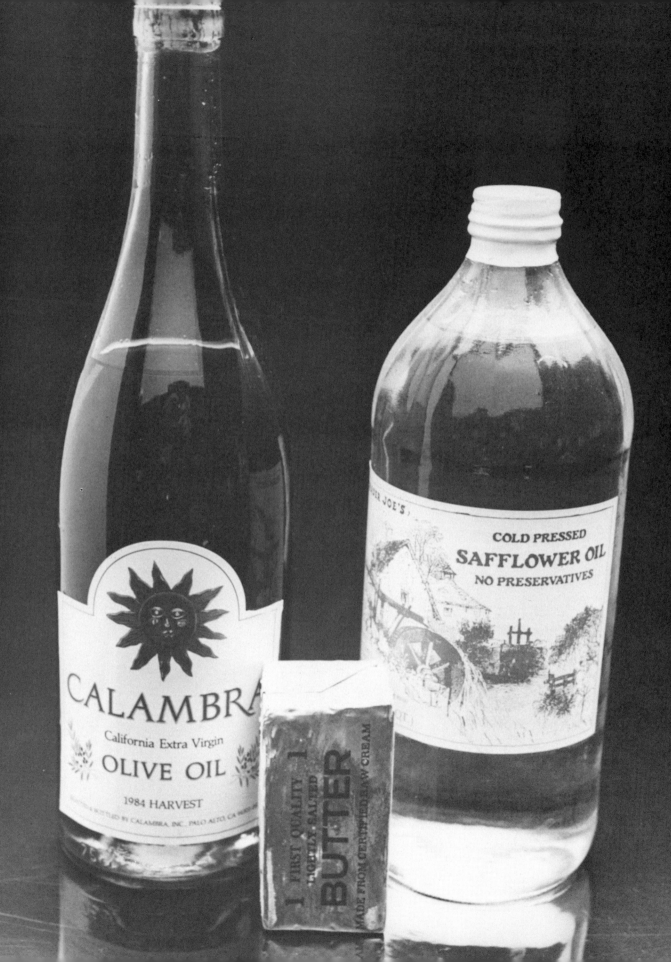

3
FATS

In modern industrial countries we have developed quite a taste for dietary fats. Indeed, the average American and Canadian consumes three to four times as many calories in fat as in protein or carbohydrate.

However, bodybuilders are tremendously conscious of the fat content of their diets. Sometimes bodybuilders monitor their dietary fat consumption to the point where they possibly cause damage to their health. But in general, bodybuilders approach an ideal caloric ratio of 60–30–10 in carbohydrates, protein, and fats.

Polyunsaturated fats from vegetable sources are a vital component in your diet. They are necessary for healthy confor-mation and function of your nerves, skin, and hair. The linoleic acid, arachidonic acid, and linolenic acid (called essential fatty acids) are necessary for proper metabolism of body fat stores. And fats are necessary for transportation and proper use of the fat- soluble vitamins—A, D, E, and K.

The saturated fats found in animal flesh, egg yolks, and milk products, however, have no useful function in a bodybuilder's diet. They do provide some of the taste found in animal protein foods, but saturated fats also provide more than twice as many calories per gram than either protein or carbohydrate. (One gram of fat equals approximately nine calories, while a gram of either protein or carbohydrate equals approximately four calories.)

CHOLESTEROL AND TRIGLYCERIDES

Cholesterol and triglycerides have been implicated in heart and vascular disease. Cholesterol is an essential dietary factor necessary for the manufacture of vitamin D in the body, formation of cell walls and nerve sheaths, and production of a variety of hormones. But excess cholesterol can be deposited as plaques in your arterial system, gradually narrowing—and even eventually completely clogging—the bore of arteries.

Very little cholesterol is required for healthy bodily function, however. Even a vegetarian diet, inherently very low in cholesterol content, will provide sufficient cholesterol for the health of cells and nerves, and production of hormones. Therefore, a diet of skinned chicken and turkey meat, fish, egg whites, nonfat milk products, grains, seeds, nuts, fruit, and vegetables will limit cholesterol intake and help prevent formation of plaques in your arterial system.

About 80 percent of the fat in a bodybuilder's diet consists of molecules called triglycerides, which have also been implicated in cardiac disease by some researchers. You can limit your intake of triglycerides by avoiding the fats found in ice cream and other junk foods.

Much has been written lately about high-density lipoproteins (HDLs), which are a beneficial form of cholesterol making up about 30 percent of the cholesterol in your diet. When you take anabolic steroids, however, you dramatically reduce the ratio of HDLs in your blood, allowing more harmful LDLs (low-density lipoproteins) to gain the upper hand.

Since the International Federation of Bodybuilders (IFBB) has instituted a program of drug testing and control that promises to cover every level of the sport, you can inhibit the loss of HDLs by avoiding use of anabolics. Using steroids even during an offseason training cycle can be an unhealthful practice in terms of HDL inhibition.

FATS AND HUNGER

Fats help to satiate feelings of hunger, so you should only adopt a low-fat diet very gradually. Jumping right into a full-scale, low-fat diet can make you ravenously hungry. But gradually reducing total daily fat consumption in weekly increments of 10–15 grams will make it much easier to adapt to the diet.

Once you have been following a low-fat diet for three to four months there will be very little temptation to begin again eating foods high in animal fats. Even a very lean cut of beef will taste very greasy and unappetizing to you.

You will find instructions for low-fat dieting in Chapter 10. With only a minimum amount of effort, you should be able to work gradually into a pattern of healthy, low-fat eating.

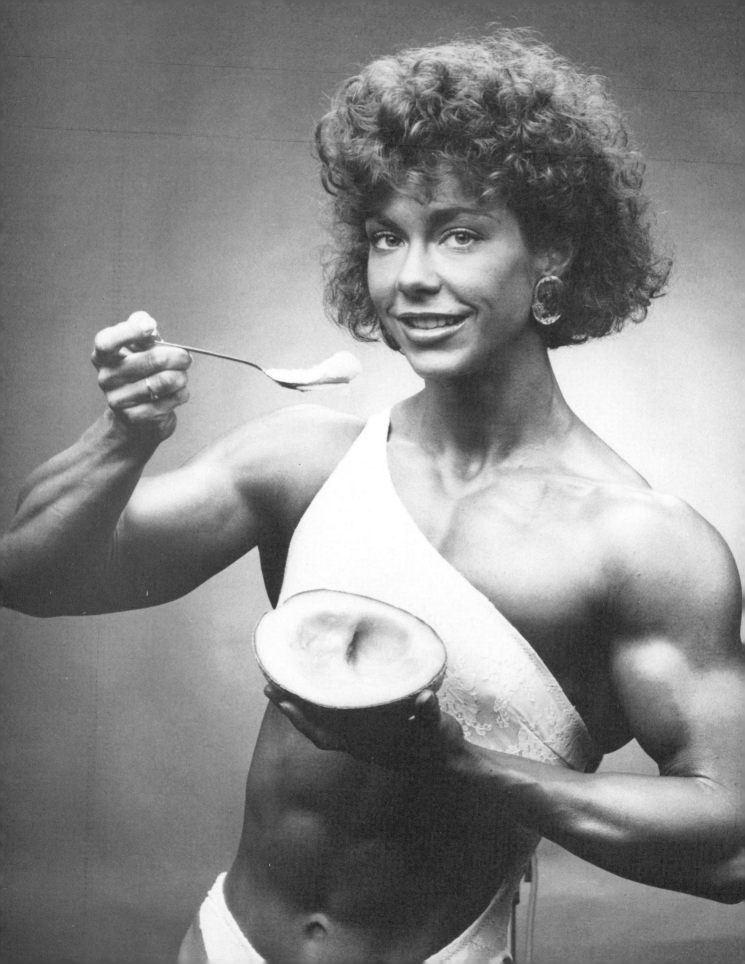

4
CARBOHYDRATES

Carbohydrate foods are a vital element in any serious body-builder's diet because they provide the fuel for forceful muscle contractions during a high-intensity workout. Indeed, correct choice of carbohydrate foods and the manner in which they are eaten can literally make or break you as a competitive bodybuilder.

Writing in *Muscle & Fitness* magazine, Dawn Marie Gnaegi (Expo Champion, U.S. Middleweight Champion) states, "Carbohydrate molecules all contain various combinations of elemental carbon (which is chemically represented by the letter C) and water (H_2O), giving carbohydrate a chemical structure of CH_2O. The energy boost you feel when you've consumed a carbohydrate food comes from breaking up the energy bonds that hold the carbon, hydrogen, and oxygen atoms together to form the carbohydrate molecule. And the amount of energy received and the speed with which that energy is released depend on the complexity of various carbohydrate molecules.

"Crucially, carbohydrate is your body's preferred source of metabolic energy. Carbohydrates yield approximately four calories of energy per gram, about the same as a gram of protein yields. A gram of fat, in contrast, yields more than twice as many calories when metabolized for energy. However, carbohydrates are more easily digested and metabolized for energy than protein, and both are burned more easily than fats."

While all biochemical evidence points to the contrary, many bodybuilders follow a carbohydrate deprivation diet prior to a show, rather than cutting back on total dietary calories in order to maintain a high degree of muscle mass while stripping off excess fat. Dawn Marie reveals, "If you are following a low-carbohydrate diet, your body will be forced to metabolize both fat and muscle protein for workout and body maintenance energy because you don't have sufficient glycogen (sugar) in your muscles, liver, and blood stream. This is why bodybuilders who follow low- or zero-carb diets prior to a show invariably end up losing disappointingly large amounts of muscle mass in the weeks leading up to a show. And they suffer grievously from the low energy reserves, depression, irritability, and general malaise that accompany limited carbohydrate diets."

Since it is possible to consume a large amount of tasty fat when on a low-carb diet, some of the best male and female bodybuilders love to follow it prior to a competition. But the men and women who successfully use a low-carb/high-fat diet tend to be ectomorphs who find it difficult to build up muscle mass and find it just as difficult to maintain that mass when cutting up. Three good examples of this type of bodybuilder are Frank Zane (Mr. America, twice Mr. Universe, and three times Mr. Olympia), Richard Baldwin (Collegiate Mr. America, Mr. Florida, twice National Middleweight Champion), and Marjo Selin (Scandinavian Champion, European Champion).

Ms. Gnaegi continues, "Glycogen is occasionally referred to as blood sugar or muscle sugar. It is derived directly from the sugar glucose that digested carbohydrates yield. When a carbohydrate-produced glycogen deficit exists in your body, muscle protein is cannibalized to make up for the relative lack of energy. Body fat and fats in your diet can also be broken down into free fatty acids for energy, but this is a dangerous process because free fatty acids left over from energy production are deposited throughout the body as stored fat, which in turn blurs out a bodybuilder's best cuts.

"It has been scientifically determined that a lack of carbohydrate in a bodybuilder's diet presents serious short-range and long-range health hazards. Over the short term, low blood

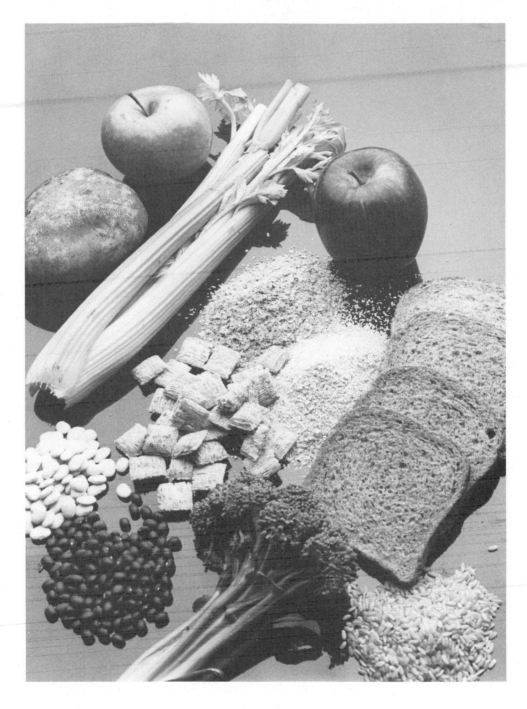

sugar levels can cause depression, low energy, slow mental function, general malaise, loss of sleep, irritability, and binge eating. Long-term low-carb dietary hazards include a deficiency of minerals in the system which in turn can cause heart rate irregularities and musculoskeletal weaknesses leading to lasting joint and connective tissue injuries."

How should carbohydrate foods be used in your diet? In order to understand the answer to that question, you must first learn the difference between simple and complex carbohydrate foods. Simple carbohydrate foods literally consist of simple chains of CH_2O molecules, which are broken down quite quickly so the energy bonds between the individual atoms can be used to supply metabolic energy. In contrast, complex carbohydrate foods consist of complex chains of CH_2O molecules, which are broken down more slowly and yield a sustained flow of metabolic energy.

"Due to their structure and ease of metabolism," continues Ms. Gnaegi, "simple carbohydrate foods yield their energy in a relatively quick burst which results in a peak of blood sugar levels. But, inevitably, the pancreas releases insulin to drive down the blood sugar levels to normal, which in turn usually yields a valley right after the peak in which blood sugar is below the normal level. Low blood sugar triggers hunger pangs, which in turn leads to the food cravings you probably feel when consuming plenty of simple carbohydrate foods.

"Simple carbohydrates are primarily found in refined foods such as sucrose (table sugar), white flour, and all of the soft drinks, cake, cookies, and so forth that are made from these ingredients. The sugar fructose, found in fruit, is also a source of simple carbs, which are often referred to as 'quick carbs' or 'fast carbs' by bodybuilders."

There are only two legitimate uses of simple carbs in a diet. The first of these is for use when carb loading following a strict carbohydrate deprivation cycle. (See Chapter 13 for a detailed treatment of carbohydrate deprivation/loading, which can add the finishing touches to an already brilliant physique.)

The second legitimate use of simple carbohydrate foods in your bodybuilding philosophy is a piece or two of fruit before a workout to provide extra training energy, or partway through the training session when energy reserves are flagging.

"An off-season junk food meal of ice cream and cookies, or pizza and a soft drink, is okay on occasion," says Dawn Marie, "but junking out should never become a regular part of your diet. But you definitely need an occasional junk food meal to preserve your sanity.

"Complex carbohydrates are primarily found in potatoes, rice, other grains, seeds, vegetables, and whole-grain pasta. These 'slow carbohydrate' foods are extremely valuable during both off-season and precontest cycles because they yield a moderate and long-lasting flow of energy. Potatoes and other starches were considered fattening foods only a few years ago, but they are now believed to be superior sources of slow-burning carbohydrates. Indeed, most of the superstars of bodybuilding base their carbohydrate intake very heavily on starchy foods.

"Allow me to use my own off-season and precontest dietary philosophies as an example of how to correctly use carbohydrates to both increase muscle mass and deepen contest cuts. As you read this, keep in mind that I'm a Libra and always seek balance in my life. I feel that any gross imbalances—either physical or psychological—will show up over the long term, so I avoid any prolonged periods of zero-carb or low-protein dieting.

"Expert nutritionists have proposed many formulas to define how much carbohydrate, protein, and fat you should include in your diet. I have intuitively arrived at an off-season formula, listed by total calories, of about 60% carbohydrates, 25% protein and 15% fats. This dietary ratio provides me with plenty of training energy, adequate protein for tissue repair and muscle growth, and a low enough fat intake to keep my body-fat levels under control.

"When I am dieting for a competition, I reduce total caloric intake primarily by cutting fats to a minimum level in my diet, plus accelerate body-fat loss by increasing caloric expenditure via an extensive aerobics schedule. You can't actually go to zero fats in your diet, because even fish has plenty of fat in it, and skinned chicken breasts have nearly twice as much fat as fish. Besides, your body requires a certain level of fat intake to maintain the health of your nerves, digestive tract, skin, and hair.

"I tend to leave my protein intake relatively constant when on a precontest diet, so when I reduce my fat intake by about two-thirds this causes the percentages of total carbohydrate calories and total protein calories to go up somewhat. So, my approximate precontest ratio of carbohydrates, protein, and fat intake is about 65–30–5.

"My carbohydrate intake year-round consists primarily of complex carbohydrate foods, and prior to a contest I eat almost exclusively complex carbo foods. I like to eat starches (potatoes and rice), whole-wheat pasta, spinach and other greens, and vegetables, particularly broccoli and asparagus.

"I consume limited simple fruit carbs in the form of bananas and apples both during an off-season cycle and when peaking. My big carb meal is usually between my morning aerobics session and my weight workout. If the carbs in this meal don't come from a potato, I'll eat mixed grains and fruit with water, or cold rice with bits of fruit mixed into it.

"If I'm low in energy despite my carbohydrate intake, I will pop 3–5 free-form amino acid capsules into my mouth and swallow them with water about 30 minutes before my workout and 3–5 more in mid-workout. I've been doing this for several years and it works incredibly well. Free-form amino acid capsules are a relatively expensive food supplement, but the benefits outweigh the cost due to augmented training energy and the fact that they build quality muscle tissue so quickly. Try amino acid capsules for a couple of weeks, and you'll feel they're worth their weight in gold.

"Your choice of foods and meal times is really just a matter of using your training instinct in a nutritional sense to learn exactly how your body reacts to various dietary stimuli. I personally prefer to eat 5–6 small meals during the day to keep my energy levels up, rather than the standard three feasts indulged in by many top bodybuilders.

"I've almost totally lost all of my junk food cravings over several years of competition, except for a rare dish of ice cream and a good, solid cookie from time to time. But as with everything else in my diet, moderation is the key in terms of junk food consumption.

"In recent years, I have followed two nutritional plans the final two weeks prior to a competition. When I was struggling to make the middleweight class limit as an amateur, I carbo depleted, but could never carbo load until I'd weighed in. After

2–3 weeks of ultra-strict dieting, carbing up even a little bit a day or two before weigh-in *will* lead to a bodyweight gain of 1–3 pounds, making it virtually impossible to make weight.

"As a professional, I am no longer forced to make weight, so I can follow a more normal carbohydrate deprivation-loading schedule. My carbohydrate intake the last two weeks consists only of rice, potatoes, and steamed broccoli. The final 72 hours, I drop out the vegetables because they bloat my stomach.

"I also cut my protein intake the last three days; then, four cups of rice and a half of a chicken breast will last me an entire day. I begin carbing up with the rice the last three days, when combined with a final-day fluid intake of only eight ounces of distilled water (with supplemental potassium and calcium carbonate) leave me ripped to shreds with an optimum degree of muscle mass for my skeletal structure.

"There will be individual variations from one bodybuilder to another, but the general formula I have presented *will* work for everyone. And the variations can soon be worked out through experimentation. Then you can use off-season and precontest carbohydrate power to develop an optimum feminine or masculine physique!"

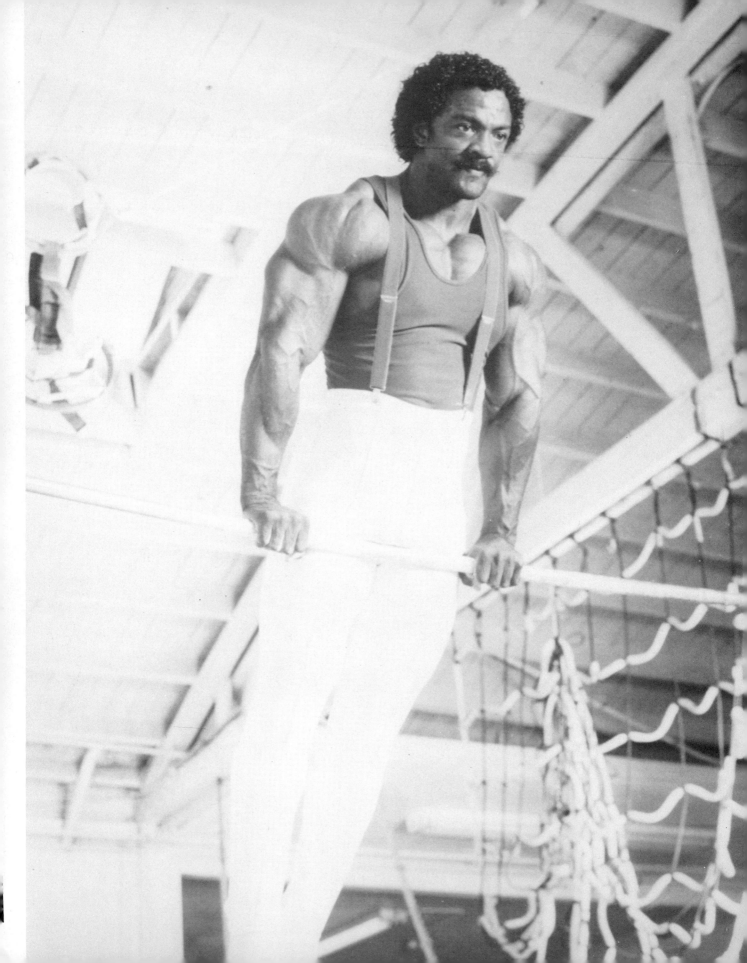

5
FIBER

Fiber, or roughage, is a component of everyone's diet that provides absolutely no food value because it is the indigestible cellulose forming the cell walls of various plants. The bran from husks of wheat, rice, and other grains is probably the best-known source of dietary fiber. Another common type of fiber is pectin, which is found primarily in pears and apples. But there are many other types of fiber found in a variety of vegetable foods.

So, why is it so important for you to consume fiber in your daily diet? At the very least, a diet high in fiber will promote bowel regularity, primarily because fiber absorbs water in the large intestine, causing the stool to be fluffy and soft. In contrast, the stool of a constipated man or woman—and there are literally millions of them in America, including many bodybuilders—is hard and lumpy. And that's the reason why it is so difficult for a constipated individual to have a normal, regular bowel movement.

You should also know that fiber in your diet speeds up the elimination of toxins through the bowels. A high-fiber diet can actually halve the amount of time it takes food to transit your entire digestive tract when compared to an individual who consumes little or no roughage.

There is also a body of scientific evidence indicating that people who live in societies like Japan, where the normal daily diet is high in fiber, tend to be healthier. In comparison to Americans, men and women in societies where fiber is a major dietary component suffer fewer diseases of the alimentary tract, such as cancer of the colon and rectum, gallstones, appendicitis, and hemorrhoids. There is also evidence that a high-fiber diet can prevent (or at least lessen) the incidence of heart disease and circulatory ailments such as varicose veins.

No one wants to die just because he or she fails to eat a particular food, right? And it simply isn't that difficult to include fiber in your off-season diet, and it's only a bit more of an inconvenience to include fiber in your precontest dietary regimen.

The easiest way to include fiber in your diet is to consume plenty of bran cereal, bran bread, fresh vegetables, fresh fruits, salad greens, nuts, and seeds. It's a simple matter to have a bowl of bran cereal with nonfat milk with your breakfast, an apple or pear for a snack, a sandwich made from bran bread for lunch, a handful of sunflower seeds for a second snack, and a salad and steamed vegetables with dinner.

During a peaking cycle, you can still have the bran cereal, salad, and steamed vegetables. Over a short period of time (six to eight weeks) this should be sufficient fiber to maintain optimum health. But as a safety margin, you can purchase cakes of pure bran in health food stores. Just be sure that you purchase bran cakes completely free of sodium, which would retain excess water in your body and blur out your sharpest cuts.

If you *do* suffer from periodic constipation, and the high-fiber diet doesn't cure the problem, you can use a natural herbal bulk laxative made from psyllium seeds. Powdered and encapsulated psyllium seeds are a very effective natural laxative. Once the capsule dissolves in your digestive tract, the psyllium acts as a sponge and expands dramatically as it absorbs water. The water-filled psyllium seeds make the stool soft and fluffy, just as it should be in order to be easily eliminated.

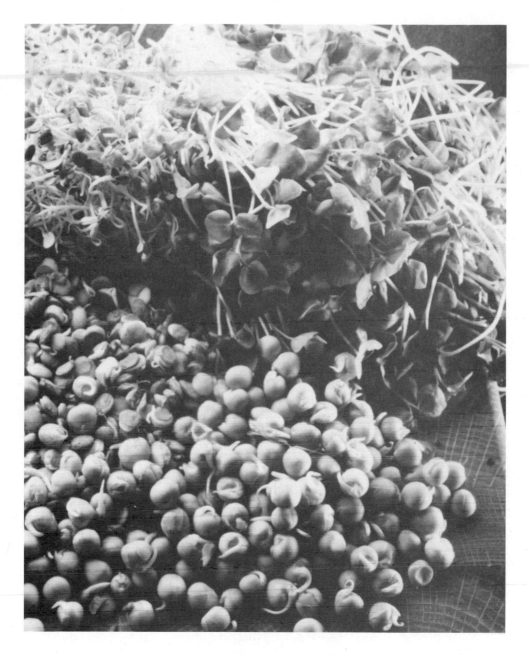

A WORD OF CAUTION

Since this book is written for bodybuilders, we assume that the vast majority of readers are healthy men and women with digestive tracts in perfect working order. If you have had chronic inflammations or other disorders of your intestines, it could be harmful to follow a diet high in fiber. Should you fall into this category, we strongly suggest that you consult with your physician prior to adopting a high-fiber diet.

Overall, however, it is our considered opinion that the benefits of consuming fiber on a daily basis far outweigh any hazzards of ingesting relatively large quantities of natural dietary fiber.

FIBER AND WEIGHT CONTROL

University experiments have shown that a high consumption of fiber might help to normalize the body fat levels of obese individuals. High-fiber foods tend to take longer to chew, which prevents you from overeating in the way many men and women do when they bolt down their food. When you eat too quickly, you may continue to gorge yourself long after your stomach signals your mind that it's full.

Along the same lines, foods high in fiber take up considerably more space per usable calorie than most other foods. Certainly, fiber that contains no calories is certainly better to have in your stomach than fatty foods like pork chops. So, if you have experienced any difficulty in losing body fat, try increasing your consumption of roughage. Perhaps you will then find it much easier to gradually melt fat from your body.

EATING FIBER

It's best to consume a wide variety of foods high in fiber, just as it's best to eat a wide variety of foods in your diet. Eat 100 percent bran cereal one day, apples the next, then pears, strawberries, watermelons, cantaloupes, honeydew melons, carrots, cabbage, green beans, corn, cucumbers, peas, kidney beans, potatoes, rice, and various types of squash.

Certainly, with the foregoing variety of high-fiber foods with which to work, you can creatively work plenty of fiber into your diet. As a bonus, most of these foods are both tasty and low in calories, so you should find it a pleasure to protect yourself from a wide variety of diseases of the digestive tract, heart, and circulatory system. Do it with fiber!

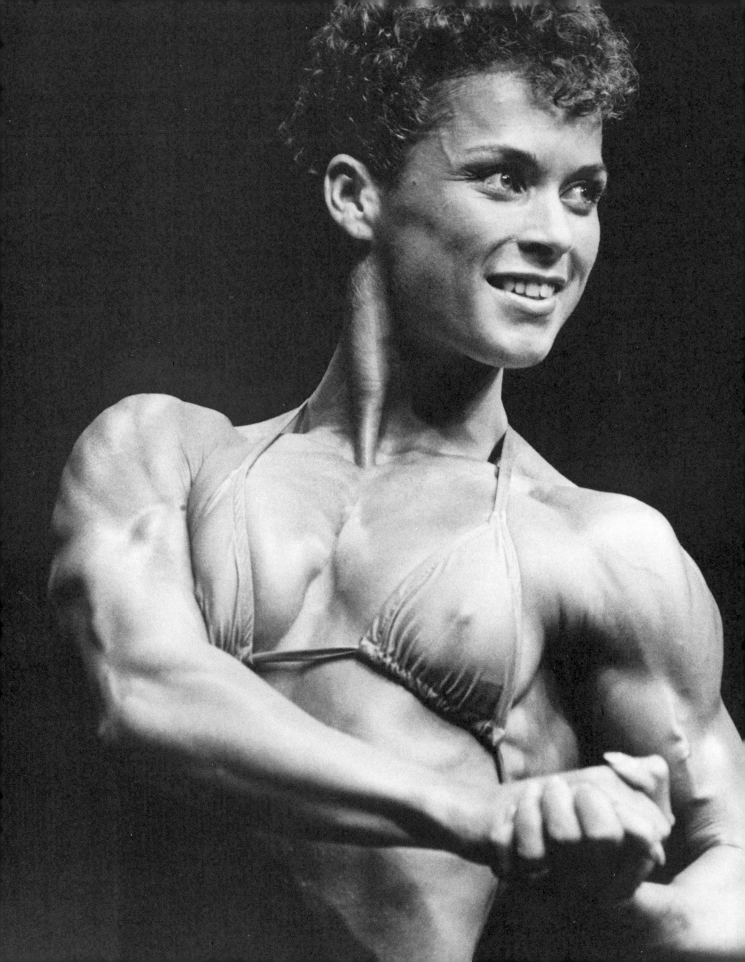

6
WATER

Despite the fact that water is a nutrient almost universally ignored by hard-training bodybuilders, it is essential to the maintenance of life itself. Roughly 70 percent of a champion's body weight is water, and 70 percent of his or her muscle weight is water as well. Blood has a very high water content, and fatty tissues also contain water although not as much by percentage as does muscle tissue. Even bone tissues contain about 25 percent water and teeth slightly less than 10 percent water.

People stranded in the desert without water and adequate shelter from direct rays of the sun cannot hope to live for more than 24 hours. But in more moderate climates with abundant sources of water, people have lived many weeks without food simply by living off of stored fat and later off muscle tissue.

Nutritionists refer to water as the universal solvent within the human body. It is involved in myriad chemical reactions within the body. Water also helps to regulate body temperature during hot days through the evaporation of perspiration. The temperature-regulating properties of water are vital to hard-training bodybuilders, so you should never be afraid to take occasional swallows of water in midworkout.

Other functions of water within your body include joint and muscle lubrication; use as a solvent in primary and secondary digestion of food; use as a vehicle for transporting toxins from your body in urine, feces, and perspiration; use as the "filler" within each cell in your body; and transportation of electrolyte minerals between cells in order to encourage powerful and sustained muscle contractions. When you grow weak and overly fatigued in the middle of a workout, chances are good that you haven't been drinking sufficient water and/or consuming enough supplemental electrolytes.

"One of the most important functions of water," maintains Dale Adrian (Mr. America and a frequent Gold's Gym habitué), "is its action as a natural cleanser within your body. Concentrations of toxic elements can be broken up, suspended in water, and excreted from your body. That's why I personally drink eight to ten large glasses of water every day. And I don't mean coffee, iced tea, or soft drinks. I only drink pure water."

WATER PURITY

If you live halfway up a mountain in Colorado and draw your drinking water from a pure, sparkling spring, you are extremely lucky. The vast majority of bodybuilders live in urban areas where the water they are supposed to drink has had enough chemicals added to it to embalm a fair-sized cat! It's little wonder that so many aspiring bodybuilders prefer to drink bottled water.

Clare Furr (U.S. and World Bodybuilding Champion) purchases bottled water, using it even for cooking. "Steve and I are very concerned with what we put into our bodies because health is just as important to us as building our bodies," Clare asserts. "Most of the year, we drink bottled spring water, but close to shows we switch to distilled water to avoid the sodium in spring water. It costs more to drink bottled water, but we both feel that the added expense is justified."

There are also excellent filtration units that can be attached to water faucets where they filter out 100 percent of the pollutants in municipally supplied water. These filters are usually made from activated charcoal, and they range in price from about $100 to more than $300. Some health food stores sell water filtration units, but you're more likely to purchase

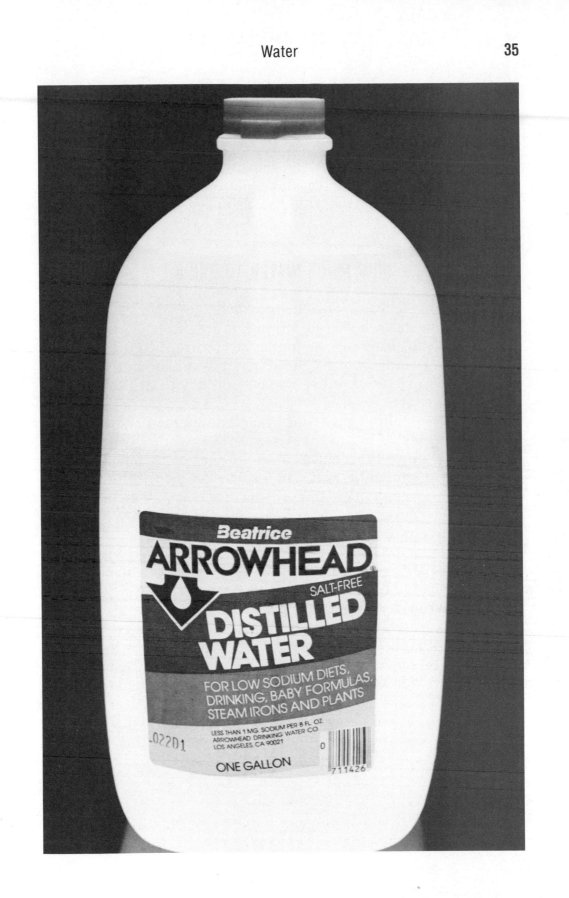

via mail order from one of the many ads for the appliances carried in health-oriented magazines like *Prevention* and *Vegetarian Times.*

Whether you use a filtration unit or purchase bottled water, we feel that it's essential for you to drink and cook with only pure water. Contaminated water can make you ill, and in rare cases even kill you. They don't give bodybuilding trophies to corpses.

HOW MUCH WATER TO DRINK

The amount of water you drink each day can vary widely according to how hot and humid it might be. And larger individuals naturally have higher water requirements than smaller men and women. Similarly, physically active bodybuilders require much more water each day than their sedentary counterparts.

Generally speaking, sedentary men and women should drink six to eight glasses of pure water each day, while bodybuilders can require more than eight to ten glasses of water each day. But the best guideline you can use to determine how much water you should drink is the sensation of thirst. Whenever you begin to feel thirsty—even if it's in the middle of a workout—stop and take a drink of water.

Dennis Tinerino (Teenage Mr. America, Mr. USA, Mr. America, Natural Mr. America, Amateur and Pro Mr. Universe) has some good advice for how to drink water during a workout: "Most bodybuilders simply gulp water from a fountain, taking in about as much air as water. And the air can cause uncomfortable stomach bloat. A much better practice is to pack a sturdy plastic cup in your gym bag, fill the cup at the fountain, and slowly drink water from the cup in order to avoid taking in any air. You'll find that this method works well. Alternatively, you can carry your own bottled water with you to each workout, a common practice among serious bodybuilders, especially during the hot summer months."

OTHER FLUIDS

Our society has placed great importance on drinking coffee, tea (hot or iced), milk, and alcoholic beverages. Each of these fluids is inferior to water, however. For example, coffee and tea contain caffeine, which has been implicated in forming lumps under the skin, particularly in women's breast tissue. Virtually every adult has at least a minor allergy to milk. And the dangers of consuming alcoholic beverages have been so well documented that only a cretin would drink wine, beer, or the hard stuff.

Since muscle tissue is 70 percent water, you will want to keep all possible water in your muscles and out from beneath your skin. We will discuss a process of body water manipulation that will accomplish precisely this goal in Chapter 14.

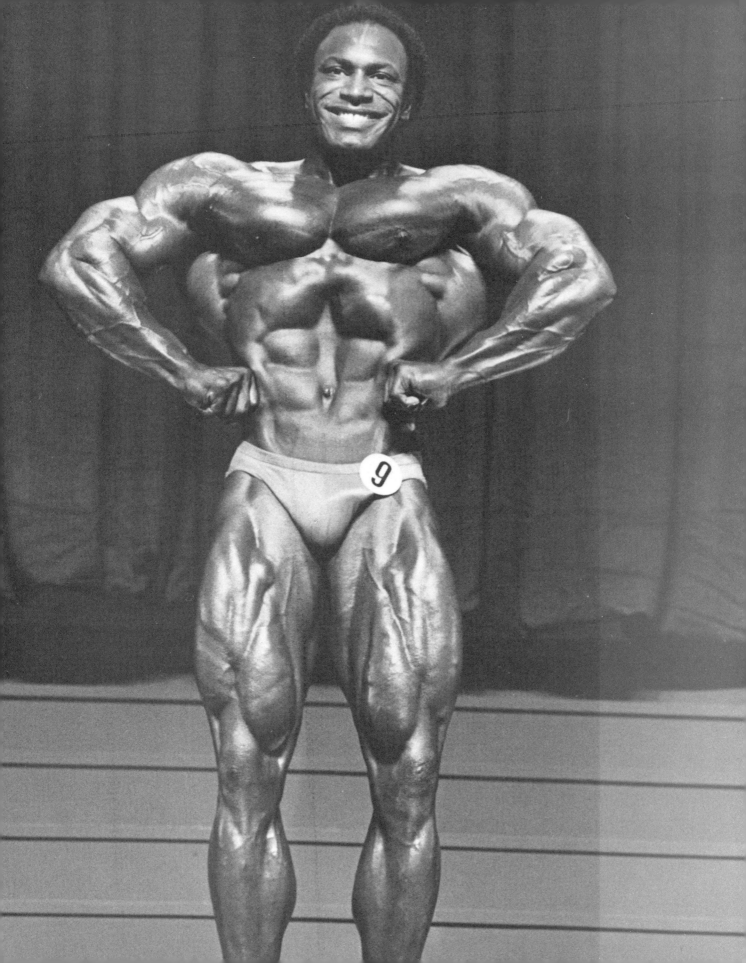

7
VITAMINS, MINERALS, AND ENZYMES

In chapters 2, 3, and 4 we discussed the three main types of caloric nutrients—proteins, fats, and carbohydrates. Now we turn our attention to three vital, but noncaloric, nutrients—vitamins, minerals, and enzymes. A balanced, healthy diet must include vitamins, minerals, and enzymes in addition to proteins, fats, and carbohydrates.

VITAMINS

There are two basic categories of vitamins—water-soluble vitamins, which are not stored in significant quantities in your body and must therefore be consumed on a daily basis to promote optimum bodybuilding results, and fat-soluble vitamins, which are stored in the human body when consumed in quantities larger than required for maintenance of perfect health.

WATER-SOLUBLE VITAMINS

By far, the most important group of water-soluble vitamins for hard-training bodybuilders belong to the family of *B-complex vitamins*. There are at least 16 individual B vitamins, most of which can be purchased in tablet or capsule form in health food stores, either individually or in complex form.

Generally speaking, you should receive more than adequate supplies of individual B vitamins by taking one to two B-complex capsules with meals two to three times per day. However, most champion bodybuilders at Gold's Gym take several different individual B vitamins each day, particularly during a peaking cycle. By carefully reviewing the benefits of each individual B vitamin and experimenting with each one, you can quickly work out the individual B vitamins your unique body requires during various stages of training and the correct dosages of each nutrient.

Vitamin B_1 (thiamine) is found naturally in milk products, brewer's yeast, beans, peas, nuts, cereals, fresh wheat germ, potatoes, pork, oysters, and calf liver. Thiamine is essential in the process of glucose reduction, which occurs in correct carbohydrate metabolism. It is also vital for nerve health and tissue growth and for proper food digestion. Without adequate supplies of thiamine in your diet, you would have low energy levels because your red blood cell count would be subpar and your blood circulation less than perfectly efficient.

Vitamin B_2 (riboflavin) is found naturally in liver, milk products, eggs, nuts, beans, and sunflower seeds. Riboflavin helps release energy from proteins, fats, and carbohydrates. A deficiency of riboflavin causes anemia because it is required for the absorption of iron from the iron-rich foods you consume. Riboflavin also promotes healthy mucous membranes and is a coenzyme that makes it possible for your body's cells to release waste products and take in oxygen, a necessity in the forceful muscular work of a bodybuilding training session.

Vitamin B_3 (niacin, nicotinic acid, nicotinamide) can be found naturally in brewer's yeast, whole wheat products, sunflower seeds, brown rice, and green vegetables. Niacin dilates blood vessels, particularly in the capillary beds beneath your skin and within your muscles, thereby increasing blood circulation. If you take too much niacin, you can feel this dilation of the capillaries in your skin as an itching sensation accompanied by flushed skin. Niacin acts with other B-complex vitamins to ensure health of the nervous system. And niacin aids in oxygen uptake in the body's individual cells.

Vitamin B_5 (pantothenic acid) is found naturally in liver and other organ meats, whole-grain cereals, eggs, green vegetables,

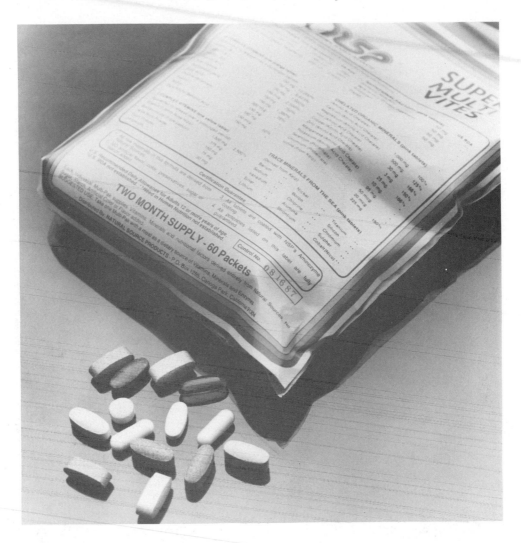

and nuts. Pantothenic acid is required for the proper use of two other B-complex vitamins, choline and para-aminobenzoic acid (PABA). By maintaining healthy function of your adrenal system, pantothenic acid promotes cell building and muscle growth. Other functions of pantothenic acid include promotion of nerve health, conversion of body fat into energy, and synthesis of antibodies to disease-bearing organisms.

Vitamin B₆ (pyridoxine) can be found naturally in liver, fish, poultry and other meats, whole-grain cereals, green vegetables, corn, peanuts, wheat germ, tomatoes, bananas, spinach, and avocados. Vitamin B_6 also comes in two other forms, pyridoxal and pyridoxamine. B_6 is essential in protein synthesis, a requirement for muscle growth. It helps the body utilize fats in your diet and aids in the formation of new red blood cells. B_6 also assists in building nerve tissue and strong bones.

Vitamin B_{10} and *vitamin B_{11}* can be found naturally in small quantities in meats (particularly organ meats), seeds, nuts, and whole grains, but B_{10} and B_{11} are also found in optimum quantities in synthetic B-complex supplements. Both B_{10} and B_{11} are necessary for muscle growth and general body growth and maturation.

Vitamin B_{12} (cobalamin) is found naturally only in brewer's yeast and animal foods such as oysters, clams, beef liver, herring, sardines, crab, and milk products. Although cobalamin is needed within your body in only small quantities, it

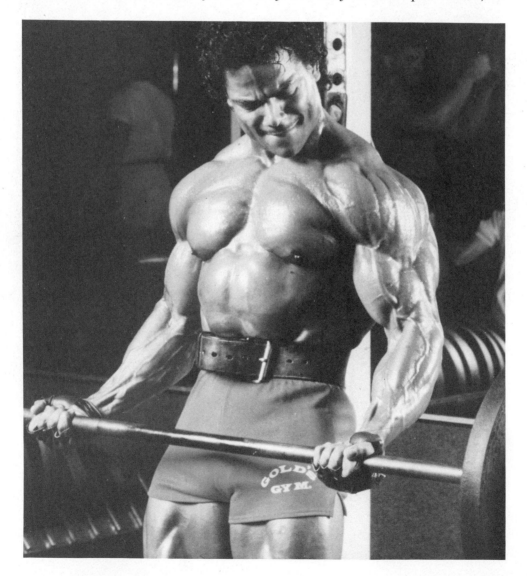

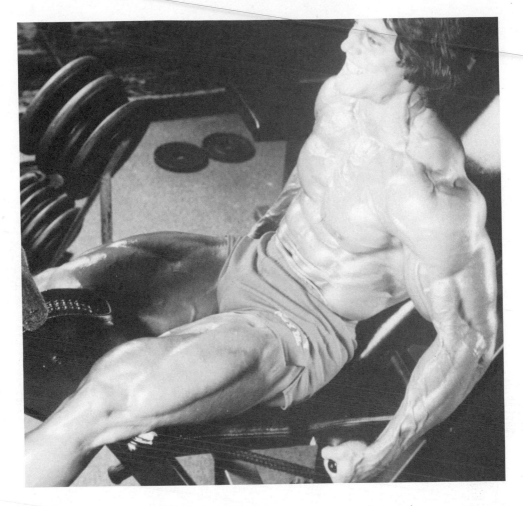

helps to form red blood cells, bone marrow, intestines, nerves, and genetic material within each cell.

Vitamin B_{13} (orotic acid) is a relative mystery in terms of natural sources and functions. Orotic acid is not yet available in supplemental form in the United States or Canada.

Vitamin B_{15} (pangamic acid) has seen wide use in the Soviet Union as an antifatigue supplement that promotes better blood circulation. Pangamic acid also helps to protect the body against environmental pollutants, stimulates immune responses, and lowers serum cholesterol.

Vitamin B_{17} (amygdalin or laetrile) is a highly controversial nutrient found naturally in the greatest quantities in apricot pits. B_{17} is the only B vitamin that is not found in brewer's yeast. While vitamin B_{17} is used to treat cancer in Mexico and other countries, the FDA proscribes its usage as a drug due to the vitamin's high cyanide content.

Choline and *inositol* are lipotrophic agents (fat burners) found naturally in brewer's yeast, wheat germ, egg yolks, and beef liver, heart, and brain tissues. Choline and inositol help to metabolize fats, particularly cholesterol. Choline and inositol were first popularized as natural agents for ripping up a bodybuilder's physique by Larry Scott (twice Mr. Olympia), Don Howorth (Mr. America) and other popular IFBB champions during the mid–1960s.

Para-aminobenzoic acid (PABA) can be found naturally in liver, brewer's yeast, whole grains, and wheat germ. PABA assists in the formation and use of folic acid and pantothenic acid. It is also important in the utilization of protein. PABA has recently been proven to have sun-screening properties and is now an ingredient in most sun screens and suntan lotions.

Folic acid is found naturally in liver, kidneys, wheat germ, dried beans and peas, and dark green, leafy vegetables. Folic acid promotes healthy nerves and builds red blood cells. It also acts in concert with cobalamin to develop genetic material within each cell.

Biotin can be found naturally in liver, kidneys, egg yolk, dark green vegetables, and green beans. Biotin helps metabolize carbohydrates for energy, and it assists in the formation of free fatty acids. Some researchers feel that biotin helps to prevent male pattern baldness.

Only small amounts of most B-complex vitamins are required to maintain optimum health and thus promote fast gains from hard workouts. But it's essential for you to understand that individual B-complex vitamins act in concert and in set proportions to one another. As a result, an excess dosage of one or more B vitamins can result in a deficiency of others.

Vitamin C (ascorbic acid) is another water-soluble vitamin. The best natural sources of vitamin C are citrus fruits, acerola cherries, turnip greens, rose hips, green peppers, strawberries, and melons. Vitamin C is a highly important nutrient with a multiplicity of functions, such as tissue repair and growth, collagen formation, bone and tooth formation, and resistance to infection and environmental pollutants. Nobel Prize–winning chemist Linus Pauling concluded that megadoses of ascorbic acid will prevent, or alleviate, symptoms of the common cold.

Vitamin P (bioflavanoids) can be found naturally in cherries, rose hips, apricots, and the white parts of citrus fruits beneath the skin and within segments of the fruit. Vitamin P is composed of rutin, hesperidin, and citrin. Bioflavanoids assist in the proper function and absorption of vitamin C. Bioflavanoids prevent bleeding gums, form healthy connective tissues, and increase resistance to infection. The best vitamin C supplements also include bioflavanoids, since the two vitamins act so closely together.

FAT-SOLUBLE VITAMINS

There are four fat-soluble vitamins that can be stored within your body and need not be taken in supplemental form on a daily basis. Some nutritionists recommend megadoses of various fat-soluble vitamins, but the FDA feels that excessive levels of vitamin A and vitamin D intake can be toxic in the human body.

Vitamin A is found naturally in the highest amounts in fish liver oil, liver, yellow vegetables, eggs, and milk products. Vitamin A is essential for healthy skin, hair, mucous membranes, bones, and teeth. A deficiency of vitamin A can result in night blindness.

Vitamin D (calciferol) is found naturally in fish liver oils, liver, tuna, salmon, and egg yolks. It can also be formed in the skin when it is exposed to sunlight. The main function of vitamin D is to assist in calcium absorption although it is also necessary for the proper use of vitamin A. Vitamins A and D are frequently found in combination in natural sources such as fish liver oil and egg yolks.

Vitamin E (tocopherol) can be found naturally in whole wheat, grain oils, peanuts, filberts, and almonds. Vitamin E is essential for a healthy heart and vascular system, as well as for proper sexual function. Vitamin E prevents blood clots within the vascular system and augments muscular endurance by conserving oxygen within the system.

Vitamin K (menadione) is found naturally in liver, egg yolk, spinach, cauliflower, and cabbage. Vitamin K is necessary for the formation of blood clots over damaged tissues.

MINERALS

There are four electrolyte minerals, three other important macro minerals, and ten trace minerals which your body requires for optimum health and athletic function. These minerals are best absorbed and utilized when they are chelated, or chemically bonded to protein molecules. Chelation turns inorganic minerals organic, which in turn makes them usable within your body.

Let us give you a good example of how well your body uses inorganic and organic forms of minerals. Health food stores sell dolomite, which is touted as a good source of calcium and magnesium. Dolomite is inorganic—nothing more than finely ground marble, the same kind of marble used for statues and interior walls of important public buildings—and we know scores of bodybuilders who have found tablets of dolomite, still whole despite the profusion of stomach acids in the digestive system, in their stool one or two days after ingesting the supplement. When calcium and magnesium are chelated, however, they can be used very readily by your body.

ELECTROLYTE MINERALS

The four electrolyte minerals (calcium, magnesium, potassium, and sodium) are essential for forceful and enduring muscle contractions. And a deficiency of these minerals—particularly calcium and potassium—can result in painful muscle cramps.

Calcium is found naturally in milk products, dried beans, peanuts, salmon, canned sardines, and green vegetables. Calcium forms healthy bones and teeth, and it acts in concert with magnesium to ensure a steady heart rhythm. Calcium also helps your body to metabolize iron, ensures strong nerve impulses to the muscles, and helps relieve insomnia and nervous tension.

Magnesium can be found naturally in nuts, seeds, whole grains, and green, leafy vegetables. Magnesium is necessary in the metabolism of vitamin C, calcium, potassium, sodium, and phosphorous. Among magnesium's multiplicity of functions are conversion of blood sugar into energy, promotion of effective nerve and muscle functions, relief of stress and psychological depression, promotion of a healthy cardiovascular system, maintenance of healthy teeth, and prevention of calcium deposits, kidney stones, and gallstones.

Potassium is found naturally in bananas, dried fruit, oranges, peanuts, dried beans and peas, meats, and potatoes. Along with calcium and phosphorous, potassium is the most essential mineral. Potassium is vital for powerful muscle contractions, maintenance of fluid and nutrient levels within each cell, and maintenance of strong nerve impulses to the muscles. Potassium relaxes the muscles, relieves irritability encountered when crash dieting, reduces hypertension (high blood pressure), aids in the metabolism of proteins, fats, and carbohydrates.

Sodium can be found naturally in table salt, milk products, eggs, fish and shellfish, meat, and celery. Sodium is often an ingredient in the sweetener used in diet soft drinks. Sodium retains water within body cells. It acts in concert with potassium to eliminate nerve impulses and powerful muscle contractions. Because sodium retains more than 50 times its weight in water within the body, most champion bodybuilders manipulate sodium intake prior to a competition to minimize body water retention and maximize muscularity. This process is described in detail in Chapter 14.

OTHER IMPORTANT MACRO MINERALS

These three minerals are required in relatively large quantities by your body for optimum health and proper bodybuilding gains.

Chlorine is found naturally in table salts and meat, as well as artificially as an additive to public drinking water. The primary function of chlorine is to combine with hydrogen atoms to produce hydrochloric acid for food digestion in the stomach. The FDA feels that chlorine prevents hepatitis and other infectious diseases although many top bodybuilders avoid chlorine by drinking bottled spring water or distilled water.

Phosphorous can be found naturally in whole grains, poultry, fish, and eggs. The primary functions of phosphorous are heart rate regulation, kidney function, and strong nerve impulses. Other functions of phosphorous include promotion of healthy teeth and gums, reduction of arthritis pain, promotion of growth and tissue repair, and metabolism of starches and fats. Phosphorous allows niacin assimilation. But phosphorous cannot be used itself unless accompanied by calcium and vitamin D.

Sulfur is found naturally in blackstrap molasses, egg yolk, brewer's yeast, yellow cheeses, nuts, whole grains, poultry, lean beef, salmon, and sardines. Several amino acids have sulfur as a constituent, and sulfur is necessary for the formation of bile in the liver, bile that is necessary for proper fat metabolism.

TRACE MINERALS

Trace minerals are necessary for optimum health and muscle growth, but these minerals are needed by your body in very small quantities. One of the best overall sources of trace minerals is sea kelp tablets.

Chromium can be found naturally in whole grains, brewer's yeast, peanuts, meat, and cheese. Chromium helps form hormones, metabolizes glucose, and activates enzymes.

Cobalt is found naturally in desiccated sea kelp. It is not that crucial of a nutrient in a bodybuilder's diet since extremely small quantities of cobalt are required for optimum health.

Copper can be found naturally in raw oysters, liver, blackstrap molasses, brewer's yeast, nuts, dried beans, cocoa, and green, leafy vegetables. Copper is essential for the formation of hemoglobin in the blood and various enzymes. Your body requires copper for proper growth and maintenance of bones and connective tissues.

Fluorine is found naturally in most animal protein foods, as well as artificially as an additive to public drinking water. Fluorine is primarily required for formation and maintenance of strong bones.

Iodine can be found naturally in sea foods, kelp, and sea salt, as well as artificially in iodized table salt. Iodine forms part of thyroid hormones and prevents goiter (enlarged thyroid). Iodine also is required for normal sexual reproduction.

Iron can be found naturally in liver, heart, red meat, clams, oysters, egg yolk, and nuts. Iron is essential for hemoglobin production. It also prevents fatigue, aids in tissue growth, and promotes resistance to disease. Iron is often deficient in the bodies of menstruating women.

Manganese is found naturally in whole grains, nuts, seeds, garlic, milk, egg yolk, and chicken. The main functions of maganese are production of various enzymes, maintenance of strength of connective tissues, protection of central nervous system function, healthy reproduction, and bone formation.

Molybdenum can be found naturally in liver, kidney, whole-grain cereals, and legumes. Molybdenum is necessary in small amounts for enzyme formation.

Selenium is found naturally in seafood, garlic, egg yolk, chicken, milk products, and whole-grain cereals. Selenium is a mild antioxidant.

Zinc can be found naturally in liver, eggs, meat, poultry, seafood, whole grains, and dairy products. Zinc is a major constituent of a large number of enzymes. It aids in the metabolism of carbohydrates, proteins, and fats. Zinc is important for optimum sexual function in men over the age of 35.

ENZYMES

There are literally hundreds of enzymes active within your body. In this section we will discuss only those supplemental enzymes that assist in digesting food, but there are hundreds of other enzymes that help build bone and other tissues, remove waste products from your body, and regulate scores of other chemical reactions within your body.

Digestive enzymes are very specific in what major nutrient they digest, so you need three different enzyme supplements to digest proteins, fats, and carbohydrates. Pepsin combines with hydrochloric acid to digest protein. Lipases help to digest fats. And amylase helps to digest starch molecules. You can find individual digestive enzymes on sale at health food stores, as well as combinations of all three types of enzymes, sometimes with hydrochloric acid included.

When you consume adequate amounts of protein, vegetable-source fats, carbohydrates, vitamins, minerals, and enzymes, you will both feel terrific and have powerful, productive bodybuilding workouts!

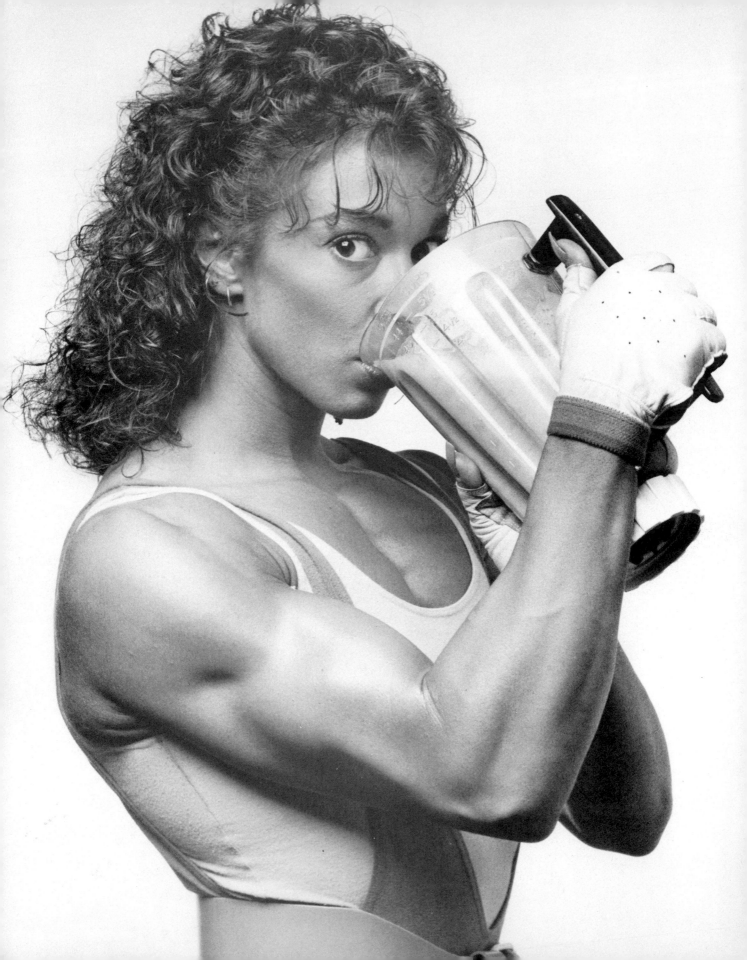

8
INSTINCTIVE SUPPLEMENTATION AND DIET

No one can deny the importance of proper nutrition in the bodybuilding process. Gold's Gym member Albert Beckles (Mr. Universe, Pro World Champion, World Grand Prix Champion) tells you why: "During an off-season cycle, training and diet are a 50–50 process in determining how successfully you add muscle mass to your frame. But prior to a competition, diet rises in importance, accounting for 75 percent of a champion's success formula, with training being only 25 percent of the battle. Prior to a show, diet helps you maintain muscle mass while stripping away all excess body fat. So, close to a show, you can really blow your chances of winning if you fail to closely monitor your diet."

As Clare Furr points out, "Diet is an even more important consideration close to a competition for women. A woman bodybuilder's physical and hormonal make-up mandate an even longer and more strict diet in order to achieve optimum contest muscularity. Women naturally have a higher body fat percentage than men, and a woman's estrogen levels further complicate the muscle-defining process."

Food supplements are an important part of almost every serious bodybuilder's nutritional philosophy. These concentrated vitamin and mineral capsules and tablets, protein powders, and amino acid liquids, powders, and capsules both provide insurance against progress-slowing nutritional deficiencies and allow a bodybuilder to elevate the muscle-building quality of his or her diet.

"Without proper food supplementation," says Gold's Gym champ Tim Belknap (Mr. America, Mr. World, Mr. Universe), "you put yourself at a disadvantage. Without supplements it becomes twice as hard to develop a significant degree of muscle mass, and it's twice as difficult to achieve peak muscularity for a major championship. I personally feel that you would be making a difficult journey to the top virtually impossible to finish if you decide not to learn how to properly supplement your diet with vitamins, minerals, and protein concentrates."

Although most bodybuilders make extensive use of food supplements, there *are* several superb athletes who have successfully prepared for major competitions using no supplements whatsoever. Two good examples of this type of bodybuilder are Clare Furr, who has placed sixth in the '84 Olympia and fifth in '85 using no supplements at all, and Ed Giuliani (Mr. Western America and one of the best bodybuilders past age 40 of all time). Eddie says, "I've prepared for the America one year using large amounts of every food supplement available and the next year using absolutely no supplements. I can categorically state that I noticed no differences in training drive, mood, or physical appearance on supplements or off supplements."

It's axiomatic in bodybuilding circles that every body is unique and has unique needs in terms of training and dietary stimuli. And this is the primary reason why you need to develop an instinctive sense of what works and doesn't work in terms of training and dietary stimuli. This is called the instinctive training principle, and you will master it by carefully equating the biofeedback signals from your body with rates of progress as a bodybuilder.

Your body requires different amounts and combinations of supplements from any other bodybuilder. And if you are just starting out in bodybuilding—or you have been training for some time with little success—you can greatly benefit from using the instinctive training principle to develop a personalized supplementation philosophy.

Actually, it's somewhat easier to master the instinctive principle in a dietary setting. Training biofeedback signals tend to

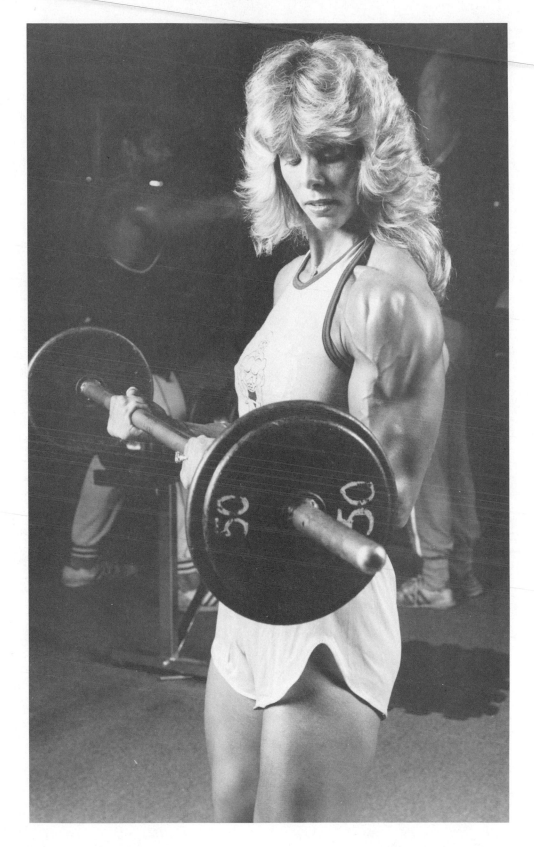

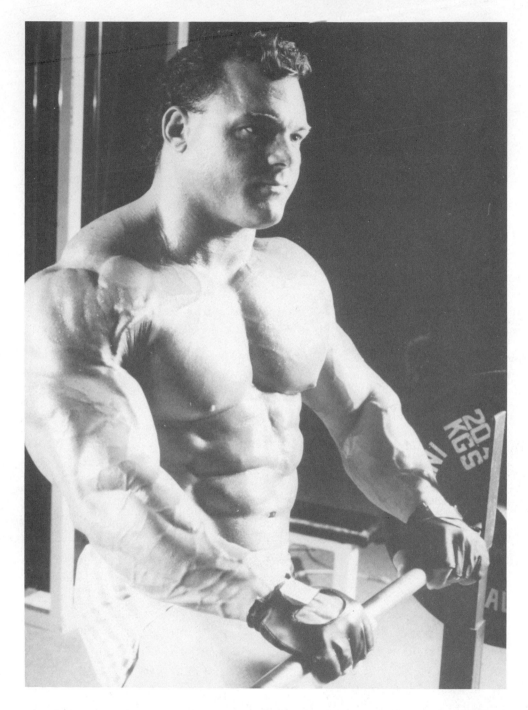

be quite subtle in comparison to dietary biofeedback. I'm sure you'll agree that it's relatively easy to tell if you are gaining or losing fat weight, if your body is bloated with excess water or not, and whether you are adding to your general degree of muscle mass.

"Other nutrition-related biofeedback signals," notes Mary Roberts (Pro World Champion, runner-up Ms. Olympia), "include relative energy levels, relative sense of well-being, relative health, clearness of skin, speed of recovery between workouts, sensations of hunger or fullness, relative ability to sleep soundly, and relative ability to relax during the day."

With all of these foregoing biofeedback data at your command, you can begin to experiment with various food supplements in your nutritional program in order to determine whether they are of value in helping you to improve your physique. The main data to observe in this context are energy levels, sense of well-being, and the rate at which you increase muscle mass and quality in your physique.

For more detailed accounts of how to develop instinctive training ability, you should read *Competitive Bodybuilding* by Joe Weider, with Bill Reynolds (Contemporary, 1984), and *The Gold's Gym Book of Bodybuilding* by Ken Sprague and Bill Reynolds (Contemporary, 1983).

Every time you experiment with a food supplement in your diet, you should change nothing else in your nutritional program. If you suddenly added three or four new supplements, for example, you wouldn't know which one was responsible for the improvement in energy or recovery ability between workouts. And you should allow at least two to three weeks, and preferably four to six weeks, to evaluate each individual supplement that you intend to introduce into your diet. Fewer than two to three weeks, and you may not allow the supplement time to kick in and affect your training and rate of progress.

If you aren't already taking one or two multipacks of vitamins, minerals, and trace elements each day, you should first experiment with multipacks. A wide variety of multipacks with high potencies of vitamins, minerals, and trace elements in timed release form are available at health food stores.

You should take a minimum of one multipack per day. But we think you'll get a lot better results—without any danger of overdosing on any one nutrient—if you take two of these multipacks per day. All vitamins and minerals, incidentally, should be taken with a meal, which increases the absorption of each supplemental nutrient. And some individual vitamins (e.g., B-complex vitamins) can cause gastric distress if taken on an empty stomach.

Chances are good that you will find multipacks to be

necessities in your diet. However, you shouldn't worry if you are among the minority who don't feel any extra benefit from multipacks. Tom Platz (Mr. Universe), for example, takes no supplemental vitamins or minerals during an off-season cycle and only a moderate amount prior to a competition. He finds that he gets adequate nutrients in the foods he consumes every day.

After you've experimented with multipacks and made a decision about whether to include them in your personalized nutritional philosophy, you should investigate the two main water-soluble vitamins, B-complex and C. I'd suggest trying B-complex first, since it is a key nutrient in the muscle-building process, both stimulating appetite and assisting in muscle tissue formation. Vitamin C assists in tissue repair among its other functions.

Following your experiments with B-complex and C, it would be logical to experiment with the three main electrolyte minerals—potassium, calcium, and magnesium—because they have a considerable effect on your workout endurance and the relative strength of muscle contractions. You might find these three minerals combined in a single tablet in some health food stores, but it's best to experiment with each one individually before trying them in various combinations. Start with potassium, and then follow up with calcium and finally magnesium.

You probably won't need to supplement your diet with additional quantities of vitamin A and vitamin D, because these oil-soluble vitamins are stored in the body, rather than being flushed out in the urine and feces like water-soluble vitamins and minerals. And vitamin D is manufactured within your body whenever your skin is exposed to the sun. So it makes little sense to take these vitamins supplementally.

One oil-soluble vitamin that you should probably run through your experimentation process is E, which plays a role in workout endurance. Most top bodybuilders take 400–1600 international units (i.u.) of vitamin E per day. You should try varying amounts of this nutrient in your own diet, using your instinct to determine whether you should be taking it on a daily basis.

These are the primary vitamins and minerals that should concern you as a bodybuilder. Of course, you can find individual B vitamins (choline, inositol, niacin, etc.) and individual minerals (iron, zinc, manganese, etc.) in any health food store,

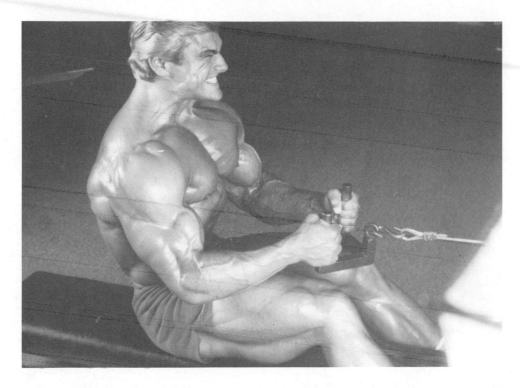

and you can eventually run experiments with these more sophisticated food elements after you've instinctively determined the value of the main food supplements just discussed.

Outside the realm of vitamin and mineral supplements, you should definitely look into protein supplementation. Most bodybuilders use protein supplements during an off-season, mass-building cycle, and many use them—particularly as individual amino acids, or amino acid complexes—during a peaking cycle. You should experiment with various protein supplements and amino acid mixtures to decide if they are of any value to you.

As discussed in Chapter 2, you probably won't receive much benefit from vegetable-source protein powders, those made from soybeans, yeast, sesame, and so on. You will, on the other hand, receive considerable benefit from taking protein powders derived from milk and eggs, foods that are among those of highest biological quality.

A milk and egg protein powder should be mixed in a blender with milk and some type of soft fruit (a banana, a peach, some strawberries) to add flavor to the drink. The resulting protein shake should be consumed either between meals, or in place of a meal that you would have ordinarily missed. We think you'll be surprised to find how much value a protein shake can have when you are attempting to gain muscular body weight.

The Porsches of protein supplements are free-form amino acid capsules and powders. Aminos cost much more than protein powders, but they are used more efficiently in the body to build muscle tissue. As a result, you don't need to take very many capsules, and the net result is similar in terms of cost to taking a protein powder.

The best times to take amino acid capsules are in mixed-amino form about an hour before a heavy workout and only arginine and ornithine an hour before bedtime. Otherwise, you can take mixed aminos during the day whenever you feel fatigued or hungry. You'll find that amino acid capsules work wonders in building quality muscle mass.

The final supplement we wish to discuss, desiccated liver tablets, is the most controversial. Some bodybuilders feel that liver helps to increase training energy, while others feel that it is at best an inferior protein supplement. You should decide for yourself whether liver tablets are of value to you in building lean muscle mass. Experiment with various quantities and check to see if they have an effect on training energy, recuperative ability, or rate of muscle mass increase.

How long should it take you to arrive at a personalized nutritional philosophy? If you follow the instructions we've given in this section of Chapter 8, it could take no more than a year of systematic experimentation to determine which supplements should be included in your dietary regimen. But the time will be well spent because you'll make much faster progress and better bodybuilding gains if you use the correct combinations and amounts of food supplements.

SUPPLEMENTATION ON A BUDGET

It is obvious to us that very few bodybuilders can afford the cost of the full supplementation program followed by many Mr. Olympia and Ms. Olympia competitors. And many young bodybuilding aspirants have very little money to spend on supplements.

If you can afford $15–$20 per month for supplements, however, you *can* supplement your diet sufficiently to improve your rate of progress as a bodybuilder. The most essential supplement is a "one-a-day" type of multiple vitamin-mineral tablet.

At a consumption rate of one to two per day (split up over two meals if you take two), a month's supply purchased at a health food store would cost $10–$12.

One of the best and least expensive protein supplements is the dry powdered nonfat milk found in any supermarket. Simply add one to two teaspoons of the powder to a glass of milk for consumption between meals. (Stir it thoroughly with a spoon, or mix it with a blender if you have one.) Alternatively, you can mix the powdered milk either double- or triple-strength with water. As long as you have no substantial allergy to milk, dry milk powder makes an excellent and inexpensive food supplement.

The best foods for a bodybuilder on a budget to purchase for meals throughout the day are chicken and eggs for protein, and potatoes, rice, salad greens, vegetables, and whatever fruit is in season for carbohydrates. Steak may be tasty to some bodybuilders, but it's expensive and is actually an inefficient source of protein.

THE FULL PROGRAM OF FOOD SUPPLEMENTS

Some bodybuilders—even men and women new to the sport—virtually live on food supplements. We know of bodybuilders who spend more than $1,500 per month on supplementary vitamins, minerals, and proteins. Oddly, however, these individuals don't seem to make as much progress as more sensible bodybuilders who spend about $50–$75 per month on proteins and vitamins and minerals.

"Most of the best bodybuilders spend under $75 per month on food supplements," notes Franco Columbu, D.C., Ph.D. (Mr. Universe and twice Mr. Olympia). "But the cost of food supplementation tends to rise for the final four to six weeks prior to an important competition. When on a calorie-restricted diet, you should take more vitamins and minerals in order to avoid nutritional deficiencies. And many of the best men and women have found great value in additional use of amino acid capsules close to a show."

Ultimately, the amount of money you spend on food supplements will depend on your budget, your relative motivation to excel as a bodybuilder, and your supplementary needs as determined instinctively. But you shouldn't worry excessively about the money you spend on supplements, because vitamins and minerals give you optimum health, which allows you to save money you would normally spend on doctor bills.

SUPPLEMENTS FOR AN ANABOLIC EFFECT

As you probably already know, the use of anabolic steroids is widespread in bodybuilding, despite specific evidence of the health dangers of anabolic drugs. So, it should come as no surprise that many bodybuilders prefer to use food supplements—not drugs—to achieve an anabolic effect.

Scientific evidence has proven that the amino acids arginine and ornithine taken at bedtime stimulates the release of human growth hormone, which rapidly increases muscle mass and power. However, your body requires three to five times the normal recommended dosages of these two aminos to significantly stimulate muscle hypertrophy. And, arginine and ornithine work better when you are also using 10–20 mixed amino acid capsules daily.

SUPPLEMENTS YOU PROBABLY WON'T NEED

You will find in health food stores many food supplements that are essentially worthless to bodybuilders. One of these is the kelp tablet, which you will be told stimulates your metabolism and helps burn off fat. In actual practice, kelp *reduces* your BMR. Kelp is a relatively good source of trace elements, but the tablets are so high in sodium that they could be dangerous to anyone prone to hypertension.

A few other supplements with dubious value are garlic capsules, raw glandulars, ginseng and other herbs, and apple cider vinegar/kelp/B_6 capsules. You will find many proponents for each of these supplements—as well as several others—but you will seldom, if ever, find a top bodybuilder who uses any of them.

HOW TO PURCHASE SUPPLEMENTS

Unless you specifically know what to look for, it's relatively easy to be ripped off when buying supplements. Some unscrupulous supplement manufacturers/distributors charge twice what a particular food product should cost, simply hoping you will believe the supplement is better because it costs more than other brands. Following are five guidelines you should use when purchasing supplements.

1. *Compare potencies per single tablet.* Some companies give the potencies for two to three tablets, which sound great compared to another company's potency list for a single tablet of the same supplement.

2. *Compare prices for supplements of equal potency.* This rule will give you the best value for your money.

3. *With mixed amino acid supplements check to see which individual aminos are included.* Some of the more expensive (and more useful) individual aminos are lysine, tryptophan, methionine and phenylalanine. Mixed aminos missing one or more of these individual amino acids are usually overpriced and ineffective.

4. *Be sure of the percentage of egg protein in milk and egg protein supplements.* The milk component is inexpensive, and the more effective egg component is very expensive. A supplement that consists of 99 percent milk and 1 percent eggs is still a milk and egg protein powder, but it's far less useful than a 50–50 mixture.

5. *Shop around.* Exactly the same food supplements can vary in price by several dollars from one health food store to another. Shop around for the best deals.

If you have several friends using food supplements, you can save considerable money (sometimes more than 50 percent) on supplements by pooling your cash and purchasing large quantities of each product at wholesale prices. Find the addresses of distributors in various muscle mags and write to several of them to determine relative discounts. Then pick the one that offers the highest quality supplements at the best discount.

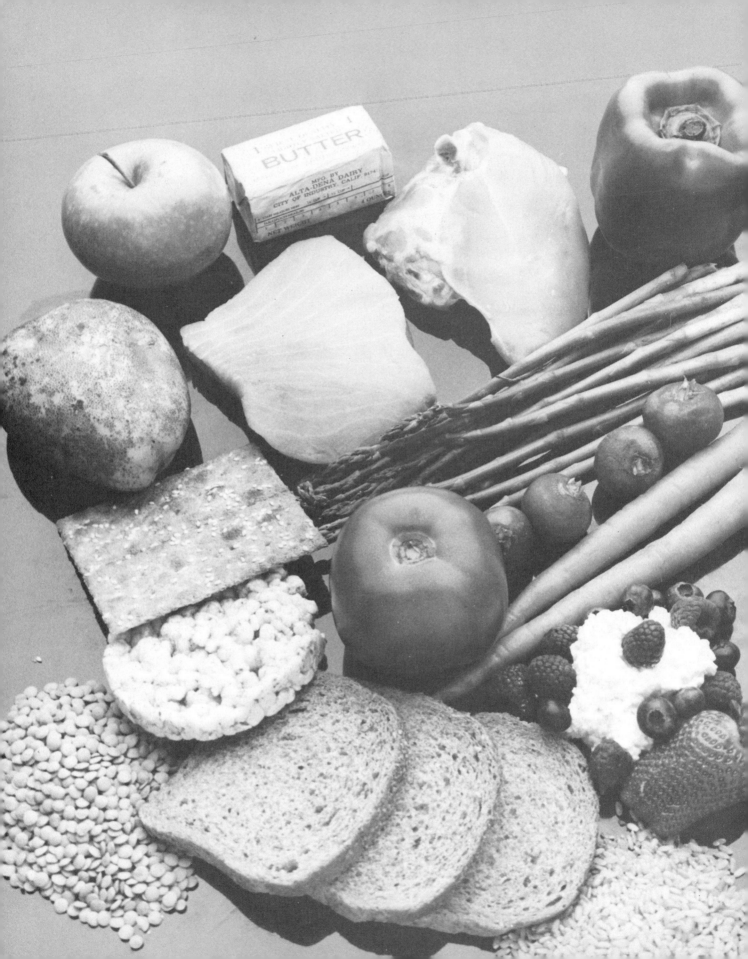

9
DIET AND EXERCISE FOR MUSCULAR WEIGHT GAIN

Without a doubt, more young male bodybuilders are interested in how to pack solid muscle on their physiques than any other aspect of sports nutrition. For example, *Muscle & Fitness* magazine, the Bible of bodybuilding, receives literally tons of mail each month, and nearly 70 percent of all the letters contain requests for dietary techniques and bodybuilding programs intended to rapidly increase muscular body weight. And there are nearly as many underweight women as men attempting to gain weight.

Nearly any man or woman in good health can gradually add muscle mass by following a heavy bodybuiding program on a regular basis and consuming healthy, muscle-building foods. But heretofore, there have been too many ineffective folk remedies for gaining muscular body weight, promulgated primarily by bodybuilders with a naturally high degree of muscle mass to begin with.

In order to gain quality muscle mass as quickly as possible, you should follow the procedures outlined in this chapter. The program definitely works because these are the same techniques used by a vast majority of Gold's Gym bodybuilders, such as Lou Ferrigno, Chris Dickerson, Lisa Elliott Kolakowski, Samir Bannout, Mike Christian, Maria Gonzalez, Steve Davis, Janice Ragain, Manny Perry, Laura Combes, Robby Robinson, and a host of other champions.

THE TRAINING DIARY

You will find that each individual dietary element reacts differently in every bodybuilder's system. In other words, forced reps work famously in building big muscles for most bodybuilders, but they are useless for gigantic Lou Ferrigno (he's 6'5" tall and weighs 270 pounds in peak condition). Therefore, you must use your instinctive training ability to determine the relative values of each nutrient in your meals. And, toward that end, it's advantageous to maintain a training/dietary diary that will reveal the long-term effects of dieting and training stimuli on your body.

A detailed discussion of training diaries in relation to the bodybuilding process and your ultimate results as an athlete can be invaluable. In our great sport, it is difficult to notice short-term improvements over a period of one to two weeks, or one to two months. However, over time, you can monitor improvement by keeping a detailed diary listing all foods consumed (including the weight of each food if necessary to more accurately determine caloric consumption); the exact exercises, sets, reps, and poundages used in each workout; and relative recuperation ability between training sessions.

There are several commercial diaries available in book stores and through mail order. One of the best of these training diaries, available in book stores or via mail order ads in *Muscle & Fitness* is Joe Weider's *Muscle & Fitness Training Diary* (Contemporary, 1982). One good mail order source for this book is Angels Camp Mercantile, Box 8, Angels Camp, CA 95222. This diary has detailed instructions on how to use it effectively, loads of training tips, and enough blank pages for six to twelve months of all-out workouts and nutritious meals.

If you prefer Nautilus training, there is a very good *Training Diary for Nautilus Exercise* (Contemporary, 1983). Or, you can try the Total Training Weightlifter's Log, available from Total Training, 6123 Sheraton Place, Aptos, CA 95003. This diary doesn't have much space for food entries, however.

Should you be unable to locate a commercially prepared personal nutrition diary, take solace in the fact that a majority of Gold's Gym members use homemade—rather than commercially produced—books. Any well-bound book with blank pages that will hold together under heavy use in a gym will do nicely. And don't forget to carry a pen or pencil along with the book so that you can make entries immediately and not forget them. The entire purpose of a training diary is to record your complete workout program and nutrition plan from day to day.

At Gold's Gym, we believe that all of the following features should be regularly included in your diary (explanations of each factor are enclosed in parentheses):

- Morning pulse rate (a spike in pulse rate can indicate an impending overtrained condition)
- Morning blood pressure (a spike in blood pressure can also indicate an impending overtrained state)
- How well and long you slept the evening before
- Mood changes (as well as what specific factors caused the change, e.g., the tension of a job-related problem, a fight with a spouse or girlfriend, etc.)
- Persistently sore joints and muscles
- All food supplements and their effect on energy and sense of well-being
- Relative energy and psychological levels
- Degree of excess water retention and the reason for it
- How strongly you finished your workout, and an estimate of what factors caused an excellent workout
- A psychological evaluation of how well you feel about yourself when you are practicing your routine (as well as how you feel onstage)
- Any aversion to training; any great desire to work out
- Enthusiasm level for upcoming workouts

The key once you have resolved any negative factors is to get into the gym and train as hard as possible without the weight of the world on your shoulders. And until you have experienced a few workouts with no distractions and with great mental concentration, you'll make muscle gains like never before.

Everyone seems to record workouts in a diary, but most bodybuilders miss the boat when it comes to recording what they eat. But without recording exactly what you eat over a period of time, you will never be able to learn the effects of various foods, caloric levels, etc., on your physique. Be different, and take the time to write down every morsel of food you consume.

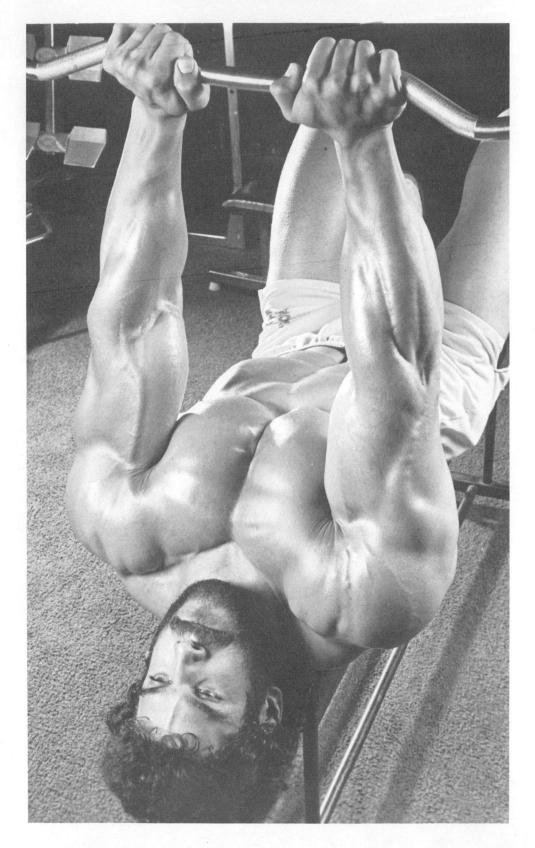

A HEALTHY DIET

Dr. Michael Walczak is well known as a physician who specializes in nutrition study and internal medicine, and he's a past president of the American College of Applied Nutrition. Dr. Walczak has tested more than 10,000 bodybuilders, film stars, and other patients during his 20 years of practice in greater Los Angeles. In the process, he has formulated nutritional programs suited perfectly to each patient's unique system and requirements.

After working for 20 years with bodybuilders, Dr. Walczak has determined one key principle: "Any bodybuilder who is in less-than-optimum health will experience great difficulty in gaining muscular body weight!"

The more you think about this statement, the more logical it will seem. Flu, for example, makes it almost impossible to recover fully between workouts, which leads to an overtrained state. And overtraining either drastically slows your progress, completely stops any bodybuilding progress, or in extreme cases actually causes a regression in physical condition.

Therefore, your mass-building diet *must* be well balanced and health-promoting to ensure optimum gains from the super-intense workouts you put in. And if you fall into the category of being a slow gainer (a nutritional program for slow gainers is presented later in this chapter), your nutritional program *must* be perfectly maintained in order for you to make gains in muscle mass.

To maintain optimum health, you should consume at least two servings per day from each of the following five food groups:

- Grains, legumes, nuts, and seeds
- Vegetables
- Fruit
- Milk products and eggs
- Meat, poultry, fish

We also recommend one multipack of vitamins and minerals each day (to be taken with a meal) as a means of nutrition insurance against undetectable dietary deficiencies. As you will recall from Chapter 8, some superstar bodybuilders consume 50 times as many vitamin and mineral units as recommended by the FDA. Using the information in Chapter 8, and your pocketbook as a guide, you can gradually work out a personalized food supplement program for yourself. But for now, one multipack per day (or two if you weigh more than 200 pounds) will be adequate nutritional insurance against progress-halting nutritional deficiencies.

THE WEIGHT-GAIN DIET

Muscle tissue contains 70 percent water, 22 percent protein, and 7 percent lipids. Lipids are largely fat, including free fatty acids, fats, phospholipids, and nonphosphorylated lipids. Therefore, the largest nonwater component of skeletal muscle tissue is protein. It's little wonder so many aspiring competitive bodybuilders use large amounts of concentrated protein powders and amino acid capsules in an effort to pack on additional muscle mass.

As long as you are training with sufficient intensity to stimulate muscle growth, the trained muscles will draw amino acids (the building blocks of protein) from your bloodstream to minutely increase the mass of the muscles you just stimulated in your workout. The bloodstream also flushes out fatigue toxins (e.g., lactic acid, carbon dioxide, etc.) and flushes into the muscles new fuel supplies (glycogen, oxygen, etc.). But as long as a bodybuilder eats well and gets sufficient sleep and rest, the crucial physiological process to a bodybuilder building muscle is having his or her system saturated with free-form amino acids. Free-form amino acids can be purchased in capsule form, or they can be derived from protein foods or protein supplements.

So when you are attempting to increase your lean body mass (muscles), you must train hard with very heavy weights *and* follow a special diet with a specialized food supplement program. Even then, gains will come rather slowly, although faster than under a normal training philosophy. Never worry about this, however, because anyone who has worked hard for a living all of his life will tell you that nothing in life worth having ever comes easily.

During an off-season cycle when you are striving specifically to bring up a weak body part and generally to increase overall body mass, diet and training are a 50–50 proposition. This means you can train all you want but fail miserably to gain muscle mass because your diet is subpar. It also means you can stuff yourself with every type of junk food imaginable, ending

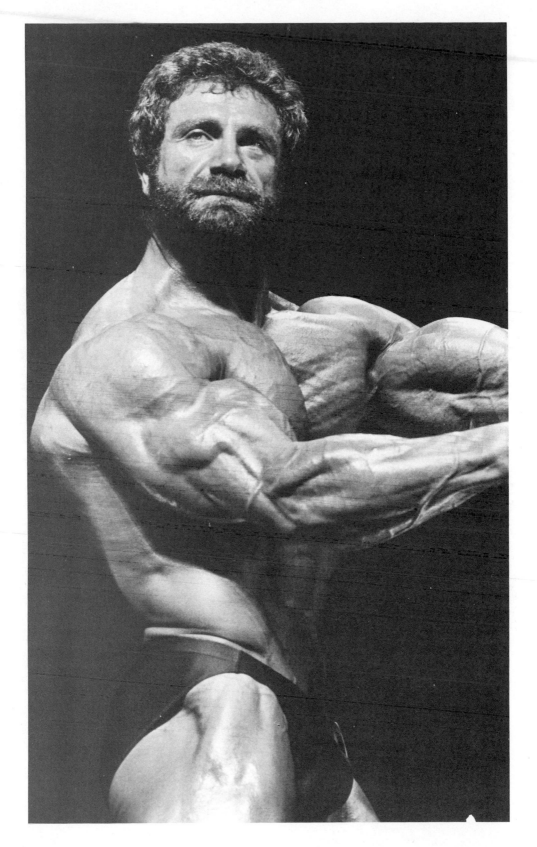

up looking like a retired sumo wrestler because you failed to train optimally.

Later in this chapter we will present three mass-building routines that you can combine with a weight-gain diet to muscle up as fast as humanly possible. There is also a large number of mass-building routines included in the also three previous books in the Gold's Gym series: *The Gold's Gym Book of Bodybuilding* (1983), *The Gold's Gym Training Encyclopedia* (1984), and *Solid Gold* (1985), all published by Contemporary Books. So, if you grow bored with any of the routines presented in this book, you will still have a wide variety of mass-building programs from which to choose.

There is one cardinal rule in bodybuilding when you are attempting to gain bodyweight: **be sure that you increase muscle mass instead of merely fattening yourself up like a pig ready for slaughter**. In this chapter, we plan to teach you how to gain pure muscle mass more quickly than under normal circumstances. True, you will inevitably gain a small amount of adipose tissue with the muscle mass, but most of your body weight gain will be in solid muscle.

For most aspiring bodybuilders, it would be relatively easy to pork up to gargantuan proportions. If you would like to include yourself in this group, start the day with a breakfast consisting of six eggs fried in butter, half a pound of bacon, all the milk you can drink and six to twelve doughnuts. Belch a couple of times and then sit down for a lunch consisting of three to four huge cheeseburgers, a mound of fries, and a large Coke. Belch two more times and eat a dinner consisting of fatty prime rib, veggies, and a large baked potato swimming in sour cream. Be sure all of your snacks consist of ice cream, cheesecake, cookies, sugar-laden soft drinks, cake, and pie, and you'll gain weight all right. Don't go swimming in the ocean, though, lest people mistake you for a whale and attempt to harpoon you.

If you're going to gain body weight, make it useful, esthetic weight rather than pork. In the immortal words of *Muscle & Fitness* photographer and bodybuilding expert John Balik, "You can't flex fat!" Any competitive bodybuilder who goes on stage with excess adipose tissue has already condemned himself to a low placing.

Muscle gains should be made slowly by consuming plenty of first-class protein foods while limiting food consumption to no more than 100–200 calories above maintenance level. As long as you follow a balanced diet and train with consistently high intensity, it will take very little additional protein in your diet to stimulate muscle hypertrophy.

The previous statement may seem ludicrous in light of the many articles you read in bodybuilding magazines about nutrition. But if you thumb through any of these magazines, you will quickly find page after page of ads for the publisher's protein powder, amino acid liquids and amino acid capsules. Therefore, it's little wonder that these magazines tout the benefits of consuming huge quantities of supplemental protein. As a result, many 200–pound male bodybuilders are consuming 300–400 grams per day of natural protein foods and supplemental proteins.

The FDA has set the AMDR for protein at one gram per kilogram (one kilogram = 2.2 pounds) of body weight. Some of the very best bodybuilders—men like Mike Mentzer (Mr. Universe), Bill Pearl (Mr. Universe), and Andreas Cahling (Mr. International), and women like Donna Lea (Ms. Canada), Dawn Marie Gnaegi (U.S. Middleweight Champion) and Dona Oliveira (American and U.S. Mixed Pairs Champion, U.S. Champion and World Games Champion)—consume either the AMDR for protein or even slightly less than the AMDR.

On the other side of the coin is long-time Gold's member, 240–pound Dave Johns (Mr. America, Mr. Universe), who habitually consumes 400 grams of protein per day, partly because he eats 48 eggs every day. A host of other champs consume comparable quantities of protein, but they fail to make good gains in muscle mass because their digestive systems are so clogged up with food that the protein foods are turned almost directly into feces, with an extremely small amount of amino acids from the food being passed into the blood stream.

One of the most rational approaches to protein consumption comes from Clare Furr (U.S. and World Champion): "In my diet I consume 1.2–1.4 times the AMDR for protein. I've experimented with all levels of protein intake. The AMDR is too low and 200–250 grams per day is excessive. So, I've chosen the middle ground."

The problem with hundreds of thousands of bodybuilders is a decision to bulk up in order to gain added muscle mass. With this theory an athlete trains very heavy primarily on basic exercises, eating like a pig and drinking gallons of moo juice. This procedure does result in a marked weight gain, a bit of it

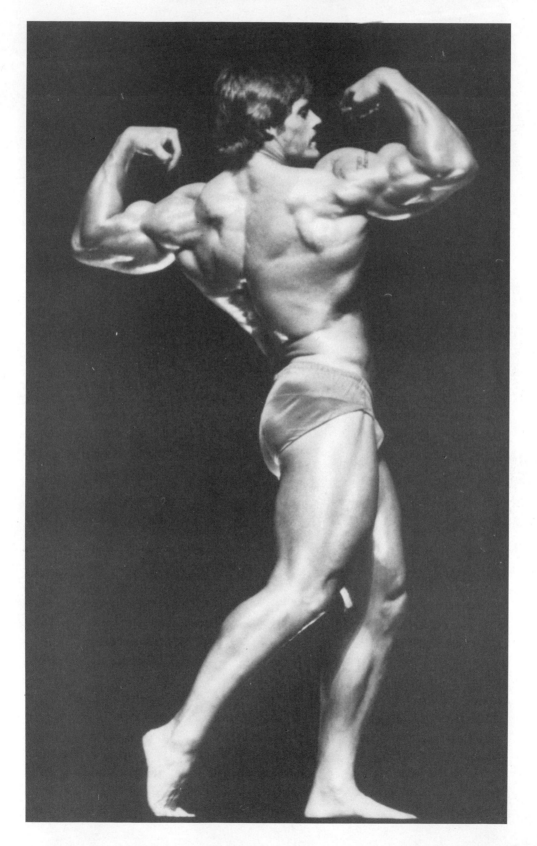

muscle mass and the remainder of it burdensome fat. Once a peak weight has been reached, a bodybuilder would initiate a strict diet and train with precontest routines in order to strip away all of the fat to reveal the "new" physique. But after starving off all of the fat, a bodybuilder would usually be lucky to gain only two to three pounds of new muscle mass.

Long-time Gold's Gym member Lou Ferrigno tells a humorous story about his experience with bulking up: "I competed in a show weighing 220 pounds, but due to my 6'5" height, I looked skinny in comparison to the guy who won. So I got out all of my old muscle magazines and researched the bulking process until I could safely feel expert enough at it to gain the 30 pounds I felt I needed to win that same show a year later.

"For nine months I trained like a madman on all of the basic exercises and ate everything that wasn't nailed down. At the end of eight months, I weighed 303 pounds and had to be careful not to bump into things whenever I turned around.

"The next four months were devoted to dieting and training down to reach a peak for the show I'd lost a year before. It was grueling work, but I managed to reach peak shape, only to lose badly again. Unfortunately, I weighed only 222 pounds, a trivial two pounds more than the previous year, despite all of the work! That experience convinced me that the process of bulking up and training down is worthless for serious bodybuilders."

Richard Gaspari (National and World Champion) has a more sane approach to gaining weight. "I've tried six-day, double-split workouts for years with few results. I've also bulked up and trained down with minimal success. My big surge during 1985 occurred because I kept my body fat percentage low all year and trained heavy while eating normal low-calorie meals."

The type of protein you consume when gaining weight is vital. The king of all the protein foods is free-form amino acids, with various protein powders also vital. All remaining first-class foods come from animal sources such as chicken, turkey, eggs, and nonfat milk products. Red meat should be avoided, and you should discard the egg yolks if you are trying to reduce or keep under control body fat percentages.

The frequency with which you eat is also crucial when attempting to increase muscle mass because your stomach can digest and make available for assimilation into muscle tissue only about 20–25 grams of protein per meal. The actual amount of protein that you digest depends on the size of your stomach, the amount of food you eat during a meal, whether you use digestive supports, and relative digestive efficiency.

Digestive supports will increase the amount of protein and other nutrients you digest. The best digestive supports for protein are various enzymes (e.g., those extracted from papaya) and hydrocholoric acid, both of which should be taken with meals. Several types of digestive supports are available at health food stores.

Since your body can digest only 20–25 grams of protein per feeding, it makes good sense to eat smaller meals more frequently throughout the day, being sure that each meal contains first-class protein. In point of fact, this is what intelligent and successful bodybuilders have been doing for many years. Rather than the two to three heavy meals an average person consumes, bodybuilders interested in increasing general muscle mass eat five to seven small meals per day. A few even eat as many as eight to ten meals per day, essentially snacking on protein foods throughout the day.

When following this plan of five to seven small meals per day, you should be sure to make these small meals nutritionally balanced. Many young male and female bodybuilders make this mistake of eating only protein each meal, which makes the diet unbalanced and can lead to nutritional deficiencies and even ill health. So, you should include grains, legumes, seeds, nuts, green vegetables, yellow vegetables, salad greens, potatoes, rice, and fruit of various types in your weight-gain diet.

Following is a suggested weight-gain menu that you can adapt to your own needs and personal food tastes:

- *Meal 1* (8:00 A.M.)—egg whites, bran cereal with nonfat milk, slice of melon, supplements, coffee
- *Meal 2* (10:30 A.M.)—tuna salad, whole-grain toast, iced tea, supplements
- *Meal 3* (1:00 P.M.)—broiled chicken breast, dry baked potato, ice water
- *Meal 4* (3:30 P.M.)—broiled trout, rice, green vegetables, iced tea
- *Meal 5* (6:00 P.M.)—protein shake with fruit
- *Meal 6* (8:30 P.M.)—roast lamb, yellow vegetable, salad, coffee, supplements
- *Meal 7* (11:00 P.M.)—seeds, nuts, nonfat yogurt

It would be folly to stick to this exact diet day after day, because variety is an important factor in formulating a healthy diet. Studies have shown that Americans tend to eat the same 12–15 foods *ad infinitum*. Unfortunately, it's impossible to receive the full spectrum of nutrients provided by nature when such a small number of individual foods are consumed. A much wider variety of food consumption encourages better health, so try to avoid eating the same meals all of the time.

Meal 5 in the example presented previously is a protein shake mixed in a blender. Here's a good recipe for a tasty nutritious protein shake:

- 8–10 oz. of low-fat or nonfat milk
- two heaping tablespoons of milk and egg protein powder
- two to three pieces of soft fruit (strawberries, bananas, peaches, etc.)

One of the easiest ways to blow a weight-gain diet is missing meals. In order to nullify this problem, simply whip up a protein shake and drink it on the run. It shouldn't take more than two to three minutes to mix one and drink it. You can also take a protein shake to work with you in a thermos bottle.

If you keep hammering on this diet while avoiding junk foods—plus train consistently hard and heavy without missing workouts—you'll slowly and steadily add quality muscle mass to your physique. It won't be easy to accomplish this, but then nothing worthwhile in life ever comes easily. Be patient.

HARD GAINERS

A very small minority of bodybuilders have so much natural talent for the sport that they make very fast gains in muscle mass. Most of the rest of us make bodybuilding gains relatively slowly. There is also a small minority of men and women who never seem to make muscle gains, regardless of how hard they seem to train and how perfectly they appear to eat.

After a few months of slaving away in the gym without making noticeable gains, many hard gainers simply give up bodybuilding in disgust. But if they modified their diet and training programs as we suggest in this section, they could begin to make acceptable progress.

Most hard gainers easily become overtrained. If they follow the same routines used by bodybuilders with great natural talent or attempt to train on a six-day split routine—which is basically all they will read about in various bodybuilding magazines—they will be unable to completely recover between workouts. This inability to recover between training sessions leads to an overtrained state, which in turn halts any progress that should result from heavy workouts. In many cases with hard gainers, a man or woman will actually regress in physical development and strength levels when overtrained.

The best type of workout for a hard gainer is a four-day split routine in which each major muscle group is trained twice per

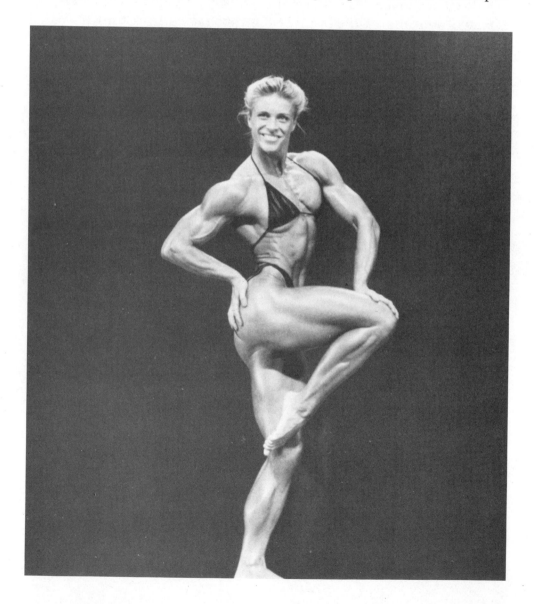

week. Here is an example of how you can split up your body parts for this type of routine:

Monday–Thursday	Tuesday–Friday
Abdominals (hard)	Abdominals (easy)
Chest	Thighs
Shoulders	Lower back
Upper back	Arms
Calves (hard)	Calves (easy)

Hard gainers should limit their total sets for each body part. For thighs, back, chest and shoulders, do no more than eight to ten total sets; for all other muscle groups, do six to eight total sets. Keep reps low (in the range of five to eight) and maintain perfect exercise form in all movements included in your routine.

It is also essential that you do almost exclusively basic exercises in your routines. Following are the best basic exercises for each muscle group:

- *Thighs*: Squats, Leg Presses, Leg Curls, Stiff-Legged Deadlifts
- *Lats*: Barbell Rows, Pulley Rows, Chins, Pulldowns
- *Traps*: Shrugs
- *Erectors*: Deadlifts, Stiff-Legged Deadlifts
- *Chest*: Bench Presses, Incline Presses, Parallel Bar Dips
- *Shoulders*: Barbell Presses, Dumbbell Presses, Upright Rows
- *Biceps*: Barbell Curls, Barbell Preacher Curls
- *Triceps*: Close-Grip Bench Presses, Dips, Barbell Triceps Extensions
- *Forearms*: Reverse Curls, Barbell Wrist Curls
- *Calves*: Seated Calf Machine Toe Raises, Standing Calf Machine Toe Raises
- *Abdominals*: Hanging Leg Raises, Incline Sit-Ups, Crunches

Always get as much sleep and rest as possible because your muscles increase in size and strength only when your body is at rest. Avoid nervous energy leaks. And avoid doing aerobic activities such as running, cycling, and swimming. All of a hard-gainer's energy reserves should be conserved for heavy bodybuilding workouts, recovery from those workouts, and muscle growth.

Follow the dietary procedures outlined earlier in this chapter, but add amino acid capsules to your diet. We suggest two to three capsules of mixed aminos between meals to encourage a positive nitrogen balance in your body. (Nitrogen is a major component of protein.) At bedtime, take two to three capsules each of arginine and ornithine, which release your body's growth factors and add to muscle mass.

Finally, keep a consistently positive mental attitude and be patient. It definitely takes time for a slow gainer to increase muscle mass, but all of the work and self-discipline will be worthwhile once you've reached the degree of physical development you seek.

REASONABLE EXPECTATIONS

How much muscular body weight can an average bodybuilder expect to pack on in one year of mass-building workouts and diet? We asked two Gold's Gym champions this question.

"If you gain five to six pounds of solid muscle per year, you're doing really well," explained Mike Christian (California, National, and World Champion). "Of course I see a lot of men add more than that, but most of their weight gain is in fat rather than muscle. And it's pure muscle that wins titles."

"Women obviously gain muscle mass more slowly than men," said Dawn Marie Gnaegi (U.S. Champion). "A gain of two to three pounds of pure muscle mass would be great over a one-year period, and it would significantly improve the appearance of a woman bodybuilder's physique."

WEIGHT-GAIN WORKOUTS

When attempting to gain weight, it's best to use primarily basic exercises in your training programs. These are the movements for large muscle groups in which you can handle substantial poundages. Basic exercises often require the use of adjacent muscle groups, such as the deltoids and triceps coming into play when you do Bench Presses for your pectorals.

We are including three weight-gain workouts in this section. The first is for relative beginners to the sport, the second is for intermediates, and the third is for advanced men and women.

WORKOUT #1
MONDAY–WEDNESDAY–FRIDAY

Exercise	Sets	Reps
Incline Sit-ups	2–3	15–20
Angled Leg Presses	4	6–10
Stiff-Legged Deadlifts	3	6–10
Seated Pulley Rows	4	6–10
Bench Presses	4	6–10
Upright Rows	3	6–10
Standing Barbell Presses	3	5–8
Standing Barbell Curls	3	6–10
Lying Barbell Triceps Extensions	3	6–10
Seated Calf Raises	3–4	10–15

WORKOUT #2
MONDAY–THURSDAY

Exercise	Sets	Reps
Hanging Leg Raises	3	10–15
Hyperextensions	1–2	10–15
Squats	6	15–5*
Stiff-Legged Deadlifts	3	8–10
One-Arm Dumbbell Bent Rows	3	6–10
Front Lat Pulldowns	3	8–12
Barbell Shrugs	4	10–15
Barbell Reverse Curls	3	6–10
Barbell Wrist Curls	3	10–15
Donkey Calf Raises	3–5	15–20

Note: Squats are performed as a half pyramid with the weights increased as the reps are progressively lowered (e.g., 15, 13, 11, 9, 7, and 5 reps).

TUESDAY–FRIDAY

Exercise	Sets	Reps
Roman Chair Sit-Ups	3	25
Incline Barbell Presses	4	6–10
Parallel Bar Dips	4	8–12
Flat-Bench Flyes	3	8–10
Seated Presses Behind Neck	4	6–10
Dumbbell Side Laterals	3	8–10
Barbell Preacher Curls	4	8–10
Pulley Pushdowns	4	8–10
Standing Barbell Wrist Curls	3	10–15
Standing Calf Raises	3–5	10–15

WORKOUT #3

Note: In this program, you will divide your body parts into three groups, training them over a three-day period. On the fourth day you should rest so that you will be fresh to begin the training cycle again on the fifth day.

DAY 1

Exercise	Sets	Reps
Incline Sit-Ups	2–3	20–30
Incline Barbell Presses	4	6–10
Low Decline Presses	3	8–10
Pec Deck Flyes	3	8–10
High Pulley Rows	4	8–10
Lat Machine Pulldowns Behind Neck	3	8–10
Low Pulley Rows	3	8–10
Rotating Dumbbell Shrugs	4	10–15
Standing Calf Raises	3–5	10–15

DAY 2

Exercise	Sets	Reps
Hanging Leg Raises	2–3	20–30
Lying Leg Curls	3	10–15
Seated Leg Curls	3	10–15
Leg Extensions	3	10–15
Squats	5	15–5*
Deadlifts	3	6–8
Barbell Wrist Curls	3	10–15
Barbell Reverse Curls	3	8–10

Note: Squats are performed as a half pyramid with the weights increased as the reps are progressively lowered (e.g., 15, 13, 11, 9, 7, and 5 reps).

DAY 3

Exercise	Sets	Reps
Roman Chair Sit-Ups	2–3	20–30
Pulley Upright Rows	3	8–12
Seated Dumbbell Presses	4	6–10
Dumbbell Bent Laterals	3	8–12
Pulley Pushdowns	3	8–12
Incline Barbell Triceps Extensions	3	8–12
Seated Dumbbell Curls	3	8–12
Standing Wide-Grip Barbell Curls	3	8–12
Seated Calf Raises	3–5	10–15

Note: if you are unfamiliar with any of the exercises listed in the foregoing three programs, you will find detailed descriptions and precisely posed exercise photos of each one in *The Gold's Gym Training Encyclopedia* (Contemporary, 1984).

All three of the routines in this section may seem rather simplistic to most bodybuilders. After all, they contain half of the total sets listed for the champs' routines in various body-building magazines. But these programs *work* because they don't overtax your energy reserves, allowing complete recovery between workouts. And they are short enough to permit you to train with maximum poundages without the problem of coping with great fatigue in the middle of a workout. But the diet and training programs outlined in this chapter *do* build muscle mass, and that's what bodybuilding is all about.

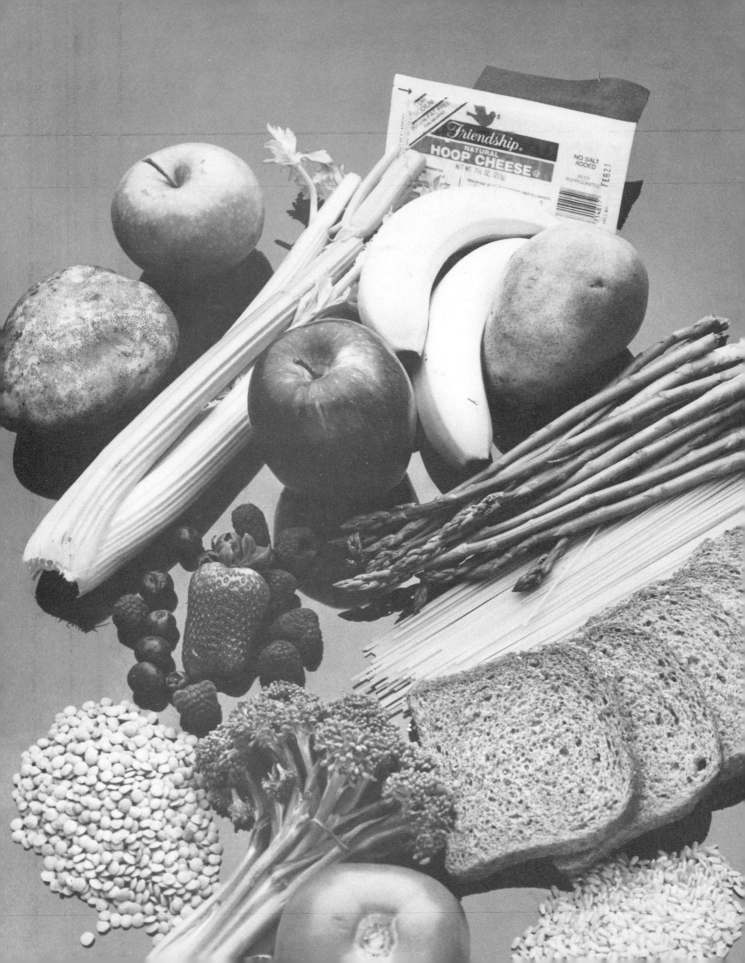

10
DIET AND EXERCISE FOR FAT LOSS

There's a big difference between dieting for fat loss and dieting for weight loss. Inevitably, at least a little muscle mass is sacrificed regardless of how scientifically you approach the dietary and training process. But most fad diets burn off muscle mass almost as quickly as body fat, which is disastrous to a serious bodybuilder.

In this chapter, we will first acquaint you with the five ways in which you can determine the percentage of fat in your body and thus the amount of lean body mass you carry at various times of the year. Then we'll thoroughly discuss the pros and cons of the two main types of fat-loss dieting—low-carbohydrate and low-fat/low-calorie. We'll also expose the fallacies of several of the more prominent fad diets. And we'll give you tips for overcoming low energy levels as you put in your weight workouts and fat-burning aerobics sessions.

Essentially, we will attempt to present all sides of the fat-loss process, giving you a chance to experiment with each method and choose the best one for you. This way, we will best equip you with the knowledge you need to burn off unwanted body fat stores without unduly depleting the muscle mass you've worked so hard to build up. And in the following chapter, we will further refine this information by presenting the best precontest diets, which will allow you to strip all of the body fat from your physique, revealing only muscle, sinew, and bone.

ASSESSING BODY COMPOSITION

The pioneer of body composition testing as a bodybuilding tool about 1980 was Mr. Ripped himself, Clarence Bass, who has taken many workouts at Gold's Gym. Through his three popular books, *Ripped, Ripped 2,* and *The Lean Advantage,* Clarence proved that frequent body composition tests can definitively tell you how much muscle you are building over a period of time, how much incidental fat you may have added to your body, how much fat you are losing on your present diet and how fast it is coming off, and how much muscle mass you are sacrificing on your diet.

Incidentally, all three of Clarence's books make fascinating reading, and they can be ordered from Clarence Bass's Ripped Enterprises, 528 Chama N.E., Albuquerque, NM 87108. All three books have extensive discussions of Clarence's experiences with body composition testing.

If you have a body composition test done each month, you can easily determine if your present training programs are effective in adding muscle mass to your physique. They will also warn you if you're getting too fat. And many of the more scientifically oriented bodybuilders—male and female alike—have body composition evaluated on at least a weekly basis to be sure they are cutting up correctly or to determine if their body fat levels are low enough. That way they know definitively that they're holding excess water if their body fat percentage is down to the super-ripped level and they still don't look quite as shredded as they should. Then, they know they must simply get the excess water out before they step onstage.

The only totally accurate measurement of body fat content is the use of a massive machine called a whole-body potassium counter. A bodybuilder sits in this machine, and the potassium ions his or her body naturally gives off are carefully counted. The correlation between an athlete's body weight and the number of potassium ions thrown off gives a totally accurate accounting of a bodybuilder's body fat amount and percentage in relation to total body weight. Unfortunately, very few whole-body potassium counters exist, and the cost of a test is astounding.

The next most accurate means of measuring body fat—and the one used by Clarence Bass and many other bodybuilders—is called hydrostatic weighing. Any college exercise physiology lab can perform this test, as can a number of the body accounting centers springing up all across the country.

Hydrostatic weighing takes into consideration your lung capacity, your weight accurately measured on a balance scale, and your weight measured as accurately as possible underwater. Since fat tissue is more buoyant than muscle, the underwater weight can be compared with your weight on the balance scale. And using a series of computations, a physiologist can give you a fairly accurate measurement of the weight of fat and lean body mass in your body, and thus your percentage of body fat.

A much more popular measure of body composition is that determined by the relative impedance of a mild electrical current run through your body. Originally, these machines didn't yield a very accurate measure of body composition because they relied on only two electrical poles, one attached to a finger and the other to a toe. And there had initially been very few correlations run between the electrical impedance machine and other more accurate measurements, such as hydrostatic weighing.

The latest machines feature four electrical poles, however, and they are much more accurate than the older models. They give very accurate calculations of body fat, muscle tissue, and body water. And there is far less hassle using this machine. You only need to lie on your back for a couple of minutes and then get a computer printout of your body composition, rather than having to be dunked in a water tank.

A fairly good home body fat measurement test can be administered with an inexpensive set of calipers used to measure the thickness of skin folds at various places on your body. By averaging up the various skin folds, you can get a reasonably accurate measurement of body fat percentage. You don't get a totally accurate measurement, but regular use of this test will give you relative body fat readings over a period of time. You can find advertisements for calipers in *Muscle & Fitness* and other bodybuilding magazines.

The final way of determining body fat is simply to look in the mirror from time to time. No judge at any competition will ever step up onstage and actually measure your body fat percentage. He or she will simply eyeball it the same as you can in the mirror. You can't go wrong when you look in the mirror and see a totally ripped-up physique.

LOW-CARBOHYDRATE DIET

During the 1960s and most of the 1970s, low-carbohydrate dieting was in vogue as the best means of achieving reasonably muscular condition. A handful of men (there weren't any serious women bodybuilders until the late 1970s) did cut calories to achieve muscular condition, but virtually everyone else limited carbohydrate intake to 60 grams per day or less whenever they felt they needed to lose excess weight, and they were relatively successful in that effort even though they invariably lost some of their hard-earned muscle mass while dieting.

During the mid-1970s, low-calorie dieting began to gain popularity, until now it is the overwhelming choice of most male and female bodybuilders. Still, there is a minority of top bodybuilders who use the old low-carbohydrate diet when trying to achieve a more muscular physical condition.

If you follow a low-carbohydrate diet, you can consume a high amount of animal fat from beef, lamb, eggs, and milk products, so this diet seems to work best for ectomorphic-type bodybuilders, or those individuals who are naturally thin and experience a great deal of difficulty in gaining muscle mass. In point of fact, virtually all of the men and women who diet on low carbs are ectomorphs.

Carbohydrate foods include anything with refined sugar or flour in it, fruit of all kinds, grains, seeds, nuts, corn, coconut, milk (although cheese or yogurt, which have the milk sugar lactose removed during processing, do not contain carbs), potatoes, sweet potatoes and, in low quantities, many other vegetables. The *Nutrition Almanac, Second Edition* (McGraw-Hill, 1984) is undoubtedly the best reference source for the amounts of carbohydrate (in grams) for various foods, as well as the amounts of protein, fat, and various other nutrients in all foods. You can also find less expensive carbohydrate-counter booklets in health food stores and drug stores.

With your carbohydrate counter and a notebook, you can keep a record of what you eat every day, noting the total grams of carbohydrate you consume. For the first few weeks of your low-carb diet, you will merely need to cut out the junk food that you've probably become addicted to during the off-season, foods such as ice cream, cookies, soft drinks, and Mom's home-baked apple pie.

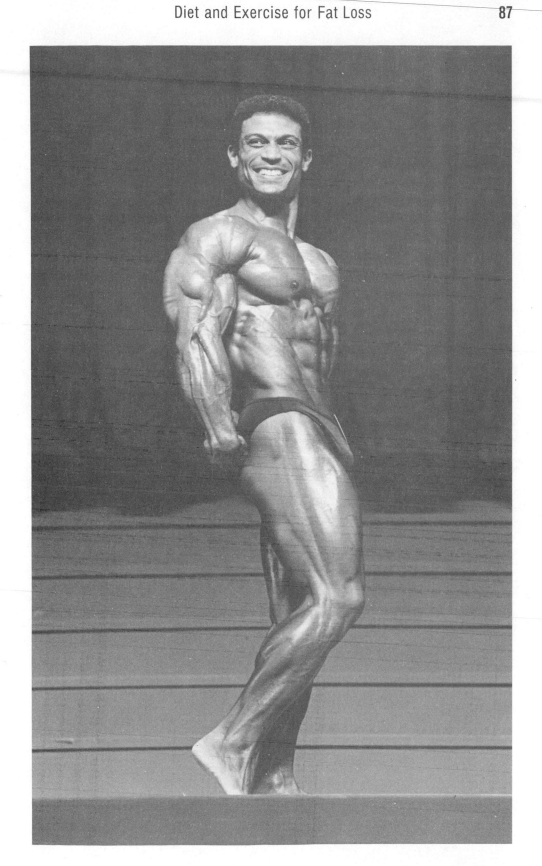

After a few days of merely cutting out the junk food, begin to limit your carbohydrate consumption to about 200 grams per day. That's a lot of carbohydrate foods, but the object of this diet is to gradually work down the amount of carbohydrate you're eating so that you don't shock your body and send yourself into an eating binge that will totally defeat the purpose of your diet.

Every three to four days, you should reduce your carbohydrate intake by about 10 additional grams, gradually working it down to the range of 50–60 grams per day for as long as it takes you to reach the degree of muscularity you're after. It is theoretically possible to actually take your carbohydrate intake down to zero—and some very foolish and desperate bodybuilders actually do cut carbs to zero—but such a practice is very unhealthy. Even at 50–60 grams of carbohydrate intake per day, your energy levels will be quite low, and you will probably feel irritable, slow-witted, jumpy, and aggressive.

A relatively tight low-carbohydrate diet would look like this for one day:

- *Breakfast*—four to six eggs fried in butter, small steak, half a cantaloupe, black coffee with artificial sweetener, vitamin-mineral multipack
- *Lunch*—steak, green beans, salad with blue cheese dressing, iced tea with artificial sweetener, free-form amino acid capsules
- *Dinner*—roast beef, green or yellow vegetable, slice or two of hard cheese, coffee with artificial sweetener, vitamin-mineral multipack
- *Snack*—hard-boiled eggs, cold cuts

Due to the high amount of fat in a low-carb diet, many bodybuilders can tolerate it quite well. However, others find themselves craving ice cream, fruit, and other sweets virtually 24 hours per day. So, for many, low-carb diets are an ordeal: these bodybuilders should instead seriously consider following a low-fat/low-calorie diet to peel off excess body fat.

Even with the high fat content of a low-carb diet, virtually all bodybuilders have fairly low energy levels when limiting carbohydrate intake. As a result, workouts can become an ordeal in which lifting even the lightest poundages is excruciatingly difficult. And because a bodybuilder is unable to train with his or her normally heavy weights, there is often a noticeable loss of muscle mass when following a low-carbohydrate diet. So, even though you might lose the excess adipose tissue you want to shed, the loss of muscle mass may not be worth the trouble of following a low-carb diet.

Low-carbohydrate diets are very poorly balanced in a nutritional sense because you can't eat fresh fruit and vegetables, grains, seeds, nuts, and other nutritional foods. As a result, your diet will be deficient in vitamins, minerals, and enzymes. To avert any chance of incurring a progress-halting, health-destroying nutritional deficiency, you *must* supplement your diet relatively heavily when limiting carbohydrate intake. At a very minimum, you should consume two to three multipacks of vitamins, minerals, and trace elements. At a maximum, you can work out your own personalized formula of individual vitamins, minerals, trace elements, and enzymes.

LOW-FAT/LOW-CALORIE DIET

By far, the most sensible, healthy, and effective diet for losing excess body fat is one in which you reduce calories below the level your body requires to maintain its current body weight. And this is most easily accomplished by reducing dietary fat intake to a minimum.

As with a low-carb diet, you should keep a nutritional diary when following a low-calorie diet. Again, you can use the *Nutrition Almanac* or other suitable calorie-counter booklets to record the number of calories in each food you consume, adding up the total each day. (Just as a handy hint, you can more easily calculate these figures each day if you frequently consume the same meals.)

It's essential that you know your approximate daily caloric maintenance level, or that number of calories required each day to maintain your body weight at an exact level. There are several complicated ways in which to calculate this figure, but the easiest is to merely multiply your bodyweight in pounds by 20. Therefore, an active 200-pound male bodybuilder would have a maintenance level of 4,000 calories per day, a 120-pound female a level of 2,400.

Once you have established an approximate daily caloric maintenance level, you can begin to gradually develop a caloric deficit each day by either cutting back on the number of calories you consume, by burning more calories through aerobic exercise (you'll learn more about aerobics later in this chapter), or by combining diet with aerobic exercise. And every time you can add up 3,500 calories that you either didn't eat, or you burned off through added exercise, you will lose one pound of useless body fat.

Through various forms of aerobic activity, you can burn up an additional 250–500 calories per hour of activity. By far, the most popular form of aerobics among both male and female bodybuilders is stationary cycling, particularly on one of the fancy cycles that's computerized to vary the work load, monitor your pulse rate, and even total up the number of calories you burned. Other popular aerobic activities include running, outdoor cycling, mountain hiking, swimming, aerobic dance, ballet and jazz dance classes, machine rowing, and various racquet sports.

"Aerobics are important for helping to keep body fat under control or to strip it off for a contest," says massive Lee Haney (National and World Champion, twice Mr. Olympia). "However, it's much easier to simply avoid a candy bar with 300 calories in it than it is to burn off 300 calories riding a stationary bike. I personally don't do much aerobics, just enough to retain good cardiorespiratory fitness. But I do keep an eagle eye on my diet. During the year leading up to my second Mr. Olympia victory, I averaged only 3,700 calories per day, and I am fairly cut on that amount of food at 260 pounds, and I'm shredded at 242 for an Olympia. If I didn't watch my diet so closely all year, however, I'd have to spend half the day doing aerobics. I'd rather spend my energy pumping iron and building bigger muscles!"

You can begin your low-calorie diet by cutting out enough fat and junk foods to get your daily intake about 300 calories under your maintenance level for the first week. And each week thereafter, reduce your caloric intake another 100 calories, until you are consuming roughly 50 percent of your maintenance level. Then simply hold that caloric intake level for as long as it takes for you to reach the body fat percentage you desire.

Since fats yield about nine calories per gram when metabolized for energy within your body (versus the four calories both a gram of carbohydrate and a gram of protein yields), it's

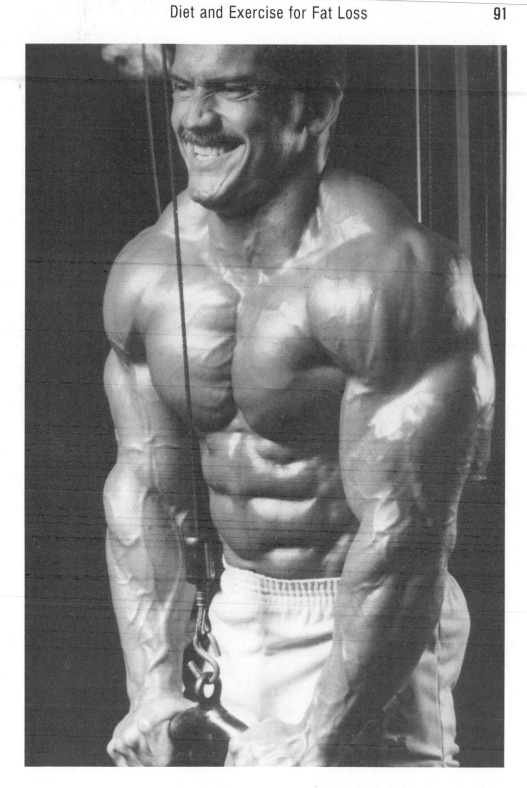

logical that you'll most easily reduce calories by cutting the fats out of your diet. Following is a list of fatty foods you should avoid when on a low-calorie diet, plus a list of foods you can use to replace those fatty foods:

Do Eat	Do Not Eat
Poultry white meat (skinned)	Beef and pork
Fish	Any canned meats (except water-packed tuna)
Egg whites	Egg yolks
Nonfat milk products	Butter and full-fat milk products
Dry baked potatoes	Potatoes with butter or sour cream
Rice	Cooking and salad oils
Green vegetables	Corn, avocados
Salads	Coconut, nuts, seeds
Unrefined grains	Refined grains (flour, etc.)
Fresh fruit	Table sugar, table salt
Dry popcorn	Mayonnaise
Vinegar, herbs, lemon juice	Commercial salad dressings

To zero you in a little more on low-fat/low-calorie eating, here are 10 additional rules you can use to amplify the foregoing lists of foods you should and should not eat:

1. *Never fry any foods.* Cooking oil is pure fat, and food fried in it invariably soaks up plenty of the oil, dramatically increasing caloric content. The most taste-pleasing way to cook poultry, fish, and other meats is over a charcoal fire. Alternatively, you can bake, grill, broil or boil meats, using various herbs for seasoning.

2. *Avoid boiling vegetables* because most of the nutrients are lost in the water used for boiling. Vegetables are best eaten raw or lightly steamed. It should go without mention that you shouldn't use oil or butter when cooking vegetables.

3. When choosing a meat for caloric content, bear in mind that fish has the lowest caloric content, poultry the next lowest, and lamb, veal, and lean beef the highest in fat. Bacon and other pork products are so high in fat that they should never be eaten.

4. Dry baked potatoes are filling and low in calories. They also taste much better dry than with butter or sour cream on them once you're used to the natural taste. Dry popcorn is also very low in calories, and it makes a great nighttime snack. An air popper is an excellent investment for any serious body-builder who likes popcorn.

5. *Avoid full-fat milk and full-fat milk products* (cheese, cottage cheese, etc.). Many elite bodybuilders avoid milk altogether because it bloats the body and skin with excess water.

6. Rather than using high-calorie commercial salad dressings, buy low-cal dressings in a health food store. Or you can use vinegar, herbs, and lemon juice as a salad dressing.

7. *Avoid sodium in your diet.* It retains more than 50 times its weight in water, bloating your body tremendously. Avoid anything with salt added to it, plus diet drinks and excessive amounts of celery, which is surprisingly high in sodium.

8. Avoid spreading butter, peanut butter, jelly, or jam on your bread, and always eat whole-grain or sprouted wheat bread. Normally it is the topping that you put on bread or toast that is high in calories, not the bread itself.

9. Cook with a wide variety of herbs in your meal plans because each new herb or spice adds a distinctive taste treat to the dish you use it in.

10. When you get cravings for certain foods not on your diet, it's best to kill the cravings by eating sweet fruits, such as watermelon, oranges, honeydew melon, or peaches.

Following the foregoing 10 rules and the lists of foods on the "do eat" and "do not eat" lists, here is a sample one-day menu for low-fat/low-calorie eating:

- *Breakfast*—egg whites (poached), half a cantaloupe, bran cereal with nonfat milk, coffee with artificial sweetener, multipack of vitamins and minerals
- *Snack*—fresh fruit
- *Lunch*—broiled chicken breast (skinned), salad, dry baked potato, iced tea with artificial sweetener
- *Snack*—free-form amino acid capsules with distilled water
- *Dinner*—broiled fish, rice, green vegetable, iced tea with artificial sweetener

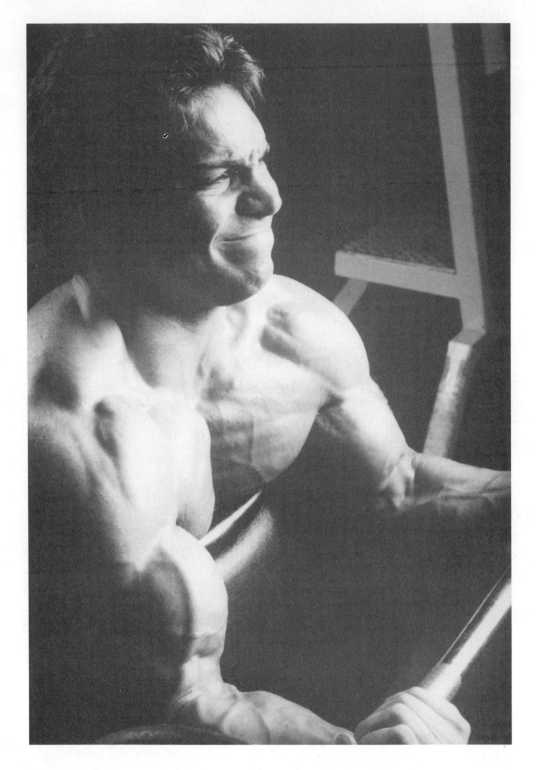

The beauty of this diet is that you'll get used to it very quickly, and any minor hunger pangs will be a thing of the past in only two to three days. And with the starch carbs included in the diet, you will feel energetic throughout the day.

FAD DIETS

Every year one or more fad diets receives great publicity—usually as a result of a book touting the particular diet—and becomes the "in" way to lose weight. Usually, these diets boast that you will lose incredible amounts of fat on them without a single hunger pang. Don't fall for this kind of hype!

Most of the fad diets are based on one form or another of low-carbohydrate eating. And once you stop eating carbohydrate foods that hold about four times their weight in water within your body, massive quantities of water are flushed from your body. This water loss looks fantastic on your bathroom scales, but it isn't an actual fat loss, and as soon as you eat some carbs and drink some water or other fluids, you'll be right back to square one in terms of body weight.

Forget about fad diets and about low-carbohydrate diets in particular. Instead, concentrate on consistently following a sensible, healthy, low-fat/low-calorie diet. In the long run, this is the only healthy and effective diet for losing weight. Eating nothing but pineapple isn't the right way to peel off body fat. Do the job right by following a balanced and nutritionally sound diet low in calories.

LOW ENERGY

At one time or another, everyone on a fat-loss diet will feel weak and low in energy. Most frequently, you will feel low in energy for the first three to five days after you initiate your low-calorie diet. But this is nothing to worry about, because it happens to everyone. The low energy during this phase is simply part of your body's adjustment to the diet.

Low energy past the first week of dieting, however, is something you should take steps to change. One of the most frequent causes of low energy during a diet is sneaking a candy bar or something else sweet into the diet. Consistently following a limited-calorie diet keeps your blood sugar levels—and hence your energy levels—on an even keel. But throw in a big jolt of sugar, and your blood sugar level quickly soars, then just as quickly crashes as soon as your pancreas releases insulin to normalize blood sugar levels in your body. So, *never* eat that candy bar, scoop of ice cream, or cookie, and you won't suffer from low energy when dieting.

Low energy past the first couple of weeks of dieting can also mean that your diet is too low in calories. If this is the case—and you are absolutely sure your low energy is a result of eating too little food—you should inch your caloric intake upward until you have a good level of energy and are still in a calorie-deficit mode and reducing your body fat. It will take a little experimentation to reach the right caloric intake level under these circumstances, but within a few days of tinkering with your food intake, you should arrive at the appropriate amount of food to both have a high degree of energy and still be able to lose unwanted body fat.

If you have a bit of trouble mobilizing enough energy for a hard workout, base most of your carbohydrate intake on starch carbs like potatoes and rice, which release energy at a low, but steady, clip. A half hour before training, have the simple carbs in a piece of fruit (apples are great) for a burst of energy to start your workout off at a quick pace. And if your energy is low halfway through a heavy training session, have another piece of fruit (oranges tend to be best at this point). Alternatively, dried fruit (e.g., raisins, dried apple chips, dried pears) can be consumed for quick energy, but avoid eating much of this high calorie dried fruit.

For a comprehensive discussion of how to improve chronically low energy levels, please read Chapter 16.

AEROBICS AND FAT LOSS

The hard anaerobic training in a bodybuilding workout burns glycogen for energy. As a result, anaerobic workouts (including hard cycling, sprinting on a track, etc.) do not burn body fat. These workouts are geared primarily toward increasing muscle mass.

"The only type of exercise that will combine with diet to strip away body fat is aerobic training," instructs Rachel McLish

(U.S. Champion, Pro World Champion, twice Ms. Olympia). "I define aerobic workouts as low-intensity, long-lasting work, such as occurs when you go jogging, cycling, swimming, taking an aerobic exercise class, or playing racquetball. At top intensity, you should be working no harder in an aerobics session than the intensity level which would still allow you to carry on a conversation. Anything faster than this, and you are training anaerobically.

"The exact timing varies from one athlete to another and from one type of aerobic activity to another, but you will normally begin to burn body fat after about 20 minutes of steady-state aerobic activity. So, close to a competition, I may do three hours or more of mixed aerobic activities. For the average man or woman dieting to lose body fat, at least 30 minutes per day of aerobic training will help enormously to lower body fat levels, improve cardiorespiratory condition, and give you a well-toned appearance. Combine high-intensity weight workouts, a sensible diet, and consistent aerobic training sessions, and you won't believe how quickly you begin looking good!"

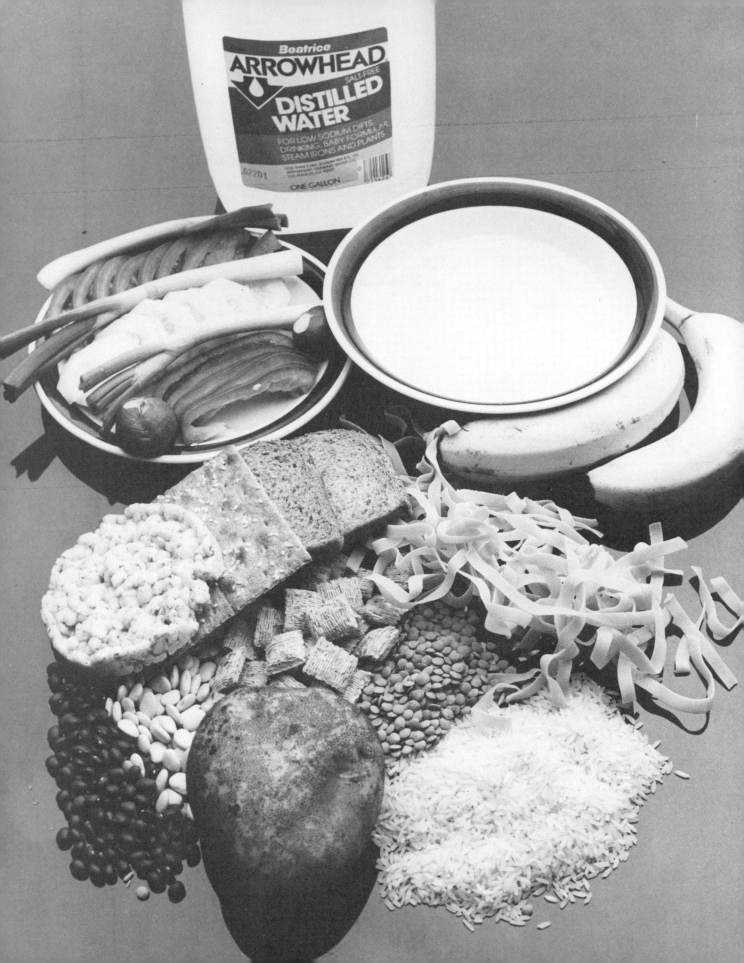

11
PRECONTEST DIET

In order to help firm up your concept of precontest bodybuilding diet, we interviewed three well-known, high-level bodybuilding champions who either currently train at Gold's Gym
or have trained there in the past. These bodybuilders encom-
pass different approaches to precontest diet. The three champions interviewed are Mike Christian (California Champion,
National Champion), Clare Furr (United States Champion,
World Champion) and Danny Padilla (U.S. Champion, American Champion, World Champion). Combined with the material
in the previous chapter, the information revealed by these
three champs will give you a good grasp of precontest diet.

LOW-CARBOHYDRATE DIETING

For many years, low-carbohydrate dieting was considered to be
the best method of achieving peak condition for a bodybuilding competition. Although low-fat/low-calorie dieting became
the most popular method of increasing muscular definition
during the early 1970s, there is still a significant number of
men and women who utilize a low-carb diet when peaking for
a contest. The most notable of these individuals is Frank Zane

(Mr. America, Mr. World, Mr. Universe, and three times Mr. Olympia).

As a serious bodybuilder, you should give each of the dietary factors presented in this book a fair trial, noting how it works to improve your body. Over a period of months—perhaps even years—you can use this system of experiments in your body lab to develop a perfect nutritional philosophy. And you should, of course, experiment with a low-carbohydrate diet.

If you are reading the chapters in this book in sequence, you already know that we discussed the low-carb diet for general body fat loss in the previous chapter. To review, it involves first eliminating junk foods from your diet, then progressively lowering the number of grams of carbohydrate in your diet, to a minimum level of 30–50 grams per day.

According to Mike Christian, "The length of time a bodybuilder should stay on a low-carb or low-calorie diet depends on how quickly and completely he or she is cutting up. If you've allowed your body weight to get out of control during an off-season cycle, you might have to limit your carbohydrate intake for three months. But if you stay within about 10–12 pounds—6–8 pounds for women—of contest condition, you probably won't need to diet for more than about six weeks.

"The length and severity of a diet is also dependent on your Basal Metabolic Rate and the amount of physical activity you undertake each day. If your metabolism is fast and you do plenty of aerobics every day, you probably won't need to diet as long or as strictly as you would if your metabolism is inherently slow and/or you fail to do significant aerobics workouts.

"I can assure you of one thing, however—you will probably

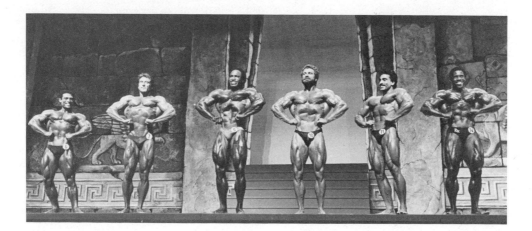

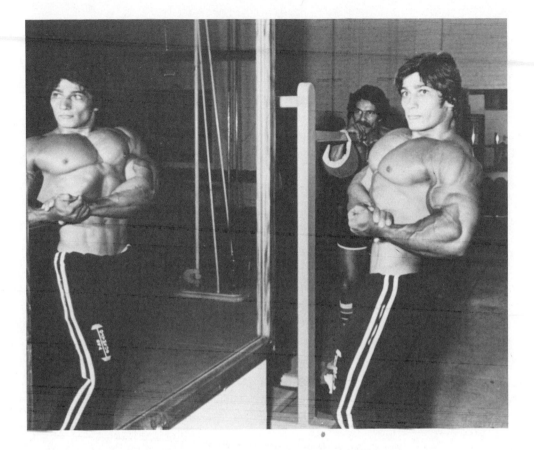

need to diet for a longer period and more strictly than you anticipate for your first competition. The average novice bodybuilder has no conception of how tough it is to attain a high degree of muscularity for a competition. That's why very few men and women in the sport have won their first competition. Usually it takes them at least one—and usually up to five—peaking attempts that fall a little short before they have developed a good appreciation of the rigors of true precontest dieting."

Clare Furr adds a word for women bodybuilders: "It's much tougher for a woman to achieve a competitive degree of muscularity than a man, because women have naturally higher amounts of body fat and slower metabolisms. Most women come into their first few shows appearing somewhat smooth, because it takes an incredible degree of self-discipline and plenty of time for a woman to achieve a high degree of muscularity.

"I've seen lots of men—including my fiancé Steve Timmreck—who do little or no aerobics and follow a diet that would fatten up most women, and who still get into incredibly muscular condition. In contrast, I have to diet strictly for three months prior to each competition, and hop on a stationary bike at least an hour each day in addition to two hours of weight work in the gym. Yes, it's much more difficult for a woman to achieve peak muscularity!"

Danny Padilla points out some of the problems with a low-carbohydrate precontest diet: "I've used a low-carb diet for contests, and I was never able to come in with an ideal combination of mass and muscularity. I might have been cut up, but my muscles looked flat and less impressive than when I'm following my normal low-calorie precontest diet.

"Among the other problems I've encountered on a low-carb diet are lack of energy for training, irritability, mood swings, lack of any sense of well-being, and awful cravings for sweets. You have to feel like you're ready for burial at times when you're peaking for a major show, so there's no point in aggravating the situation by excluding carbos from your diet. And I don't think there's any question that a low-carbohydrate diet has a negative effect on general health."

LOW-CALORIE DIETING

The vast majority of top bodybuilders follow a low-fat and low-calorie diet. By maintaining a deficit of 300–500 calories per day while eating plenty of complex and simple carbohydrates and a moderate amount of protein, you can safely and efficiently rip up your physique for a competition. This type of diet is presented in chapter 10.

As with a low-carbohydrate diet, you will probably find that you need to diet for a longer period of time at a caloric deficit to achieve optimum onstage muscularity. And you'll require regular, long-lasting aerobic workouts in addition to your normal in-the-gym sessions in order to strip away all of the excess fat to reveal every possible muscular detail. But other than these minor changes, your precontest diet will not be significantly different than the type of weight-loss diets most average people follow.

A PRITIKENESQUE APPROACH

Danny Padilla has worked at the Pritiken Center in Santa Monica, California, and his experiences have led him to adopt a modification of Nathan Pritiken's popular nutritional program. He says, "I have learned that I feel and look better in body-building terms when I severely curtail animal foods in my diet. I don't seem to need more than the AMDR in protein, which works out to about 85–90 grams per day for my body. I can build muscle tissue on that amount of protein, and I seem to recover between workouts much more rapidly when I'm not eating much meat. And, I maintain a low percentage of body fat year-round on Pritiken's diet.

"My diet in the off-season and prior to a competition consists of a limited amount of fish, plenty of amino acid capsules, raw vegetables, grains, legumes, and fruit. And as a competition approaches, I simply reduce the quantities of each food as an effective means of reducing my total caloric intake each day. In conjunction with two to three hours per day of cycling, this type of diet allows me to retain a high degree of lean body mass while stripping off all visible body fat.

"The wonder of this diet to me is the amount of workout energy I have and the great sense of well-being. And I am confident that my diet is reducing any chance of my dying from coronary disease. It's an easy diet to follow, merely Pritiken's basic diet with amino acid capsules added. I'm confident that virtually everyone would be a better body-builder if they gave my diet a good tryout."

THE MEAT, WATER, AND EGG DIET

This is an extreme version of the low-carb diet that was tremendously popular during the late 1960s and early 1970s. It still survives, even though it is now followed by a minority of somewhat misguided bodybuilders.

With this diet, you consume only meat, water, and whole eggs, with the possible exception of a small green salad once a day. Michael Walczak, M.D., one of the best-known bodybuild-ing physicians and nutritionists, abhors the meat, water, and egg diet. "It's tremendously unhealthy and ineffective," he asserts. "Bodybuilders who follow this diet end up wishing they were dead, and they usually squander all of their hard-earned off-season muscle mass on such a diet. But you wouldn't believe how fanatically loyal some people are to the diet.

"When I encounter patients who have been on the meat, water, and egg diet, my advice is to start consuming one piece of fruit and one vegetable dish each day. And when bodybuilders begin eating a little fruit and some vegetables, their physiques undergo a transformation. They fill out and begin to look healthy again, and they do this while continuing to reduce body fat stores.

"I only give this bit of advice to the hard-core proponents of the meat, water, and egg diet. Even with the fruit and vegetable each day, it's not a healthy diet. You would be far better off following a healthy, balanced diet that is low in total calories. You'll end up being in greater health and will have a much better overall degree of muscularity on a healthy, balanced, low-calorie diet."

WHEN YOU CAN'T CUT UP

There are a number of bodybuilders who enter show after show with physiques a bit deficient in muscularity. In most cases these men and women fall short of success because they cheat on their diets and/or fail to do sufficient aerobics. In a word, they're lazy, and they pay for it.

There *are* a few bodybuilders who can't seem to get completely cut up, regardless of how hard they diet and how many hours of aerobic training they do each day. In such a case, we recommend that you make an appointment with your physician for a thyroid function test. A few bodybuilders fail to get ripped up because they have deficient metabolisms. And this problem is correctable; you simply need to take thyroid tablets each morning to improve thyroid function.

If you have normal thyroid function and still can't cut up, you'll just have to tighten the screws on your precontest diet, consuming progressively fewer and fewer calories until you get the job done. No one ever promised it would be easy to win a bodybuilding competition. Dig in and do two aerobics sessions

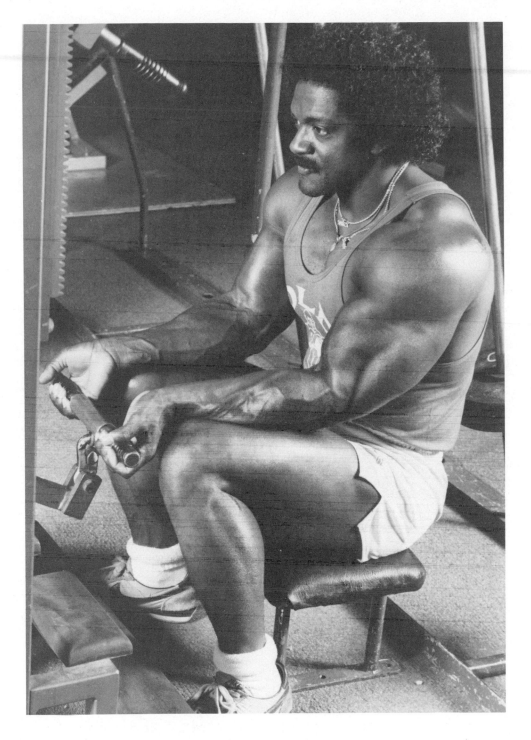

each day rather than one. Dig in and diet progressively more strictly, and sooner or later you'll develop the correct formula for achieving optimum onstage muscularity.

FINE TUNING

It's been said that bodybuilders are like orchestra conductors during a peaking cycle. They must modulate a wide range of variables—diet, aerobics, weight workouts, posing, etc.—to achieve perfect onstage condition. Implicit in this statement is the notion that plenty of fine tuning goes on in the days leading up to a competition.

With the experience you gain from peaking several times, you will develop checkpoints at one-week intervals for six to ten weeks leading up to a competition, and one-day intervals for the final week. You will soon understand precisely how you should appear at each checkpoint. Then you can reduce calories and/or increase aerobic activity if you are coming up short of the condition you wish to achieve, and you can eat more and/or do less aerobics if you're beginning to peak a little too early.

This is where the fine-tuning of your diet comes into play. With sufficient experience—gained only when you are careful to keep mental and/or graphic notes of how you appear at various checkpoints—you will be able to adjust your caloric intake upward or downward by exactly the appropriate number of calories. And once you reach this point, you will have greatly increased chances of winning your next competition.

GOING FLAT

Most bodybuilders feel they must periodically train and diet specifically to gain muscle mass, then train and diet specifically to achieve peak muscularity while retaining the muscle mass that was developed during an off-season cycle. This is really the only way you can combine maximum muscle mass with optimum definition for each competition.

Many bodybuilders get trophy-crazy at some point in their careers, peaking for many consecutive shows over a long period of time. And they pay the price for this trophy hunger by flattening out and looking as stringy as a scrawny turkey.

Therefore, we offer you this advice: compete no more often than twice per year. If you keep your body fat stores under control during a four- to nine-month off-season cycle, you can easily get into shape in two or three months for any competition. With only one or two peaks, it becomes more important to be in top shape each competition because it will be six months to a year before you compete another time. And this is the best way to achieve total muscularity combined with great muscle mass.

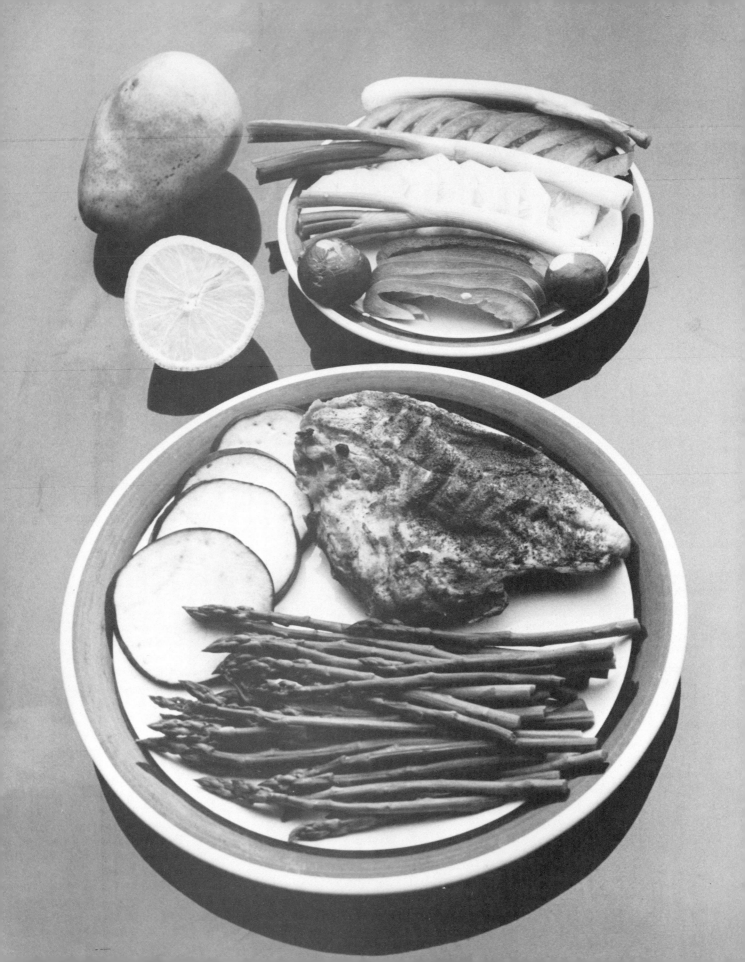

12
EATING OUT SAFELY

Consistency is the hallmark of any successful bodybuilder's diet, particularly during a peaking cycle. It's acceptable to indulge in a fast food meal once a week during the off-season, but any deviation from an optimum precontest diet can be fatal to your chances of winning a major title.

No one wants to be a drudge when peaking for a contest—and it's impossible to eat at home all of the time—so it's important for us to discuss how to eat in restaurants without fear of compromising your competitive condition. And since you will travel far from home for most of your competitions, we will also tell you in this chapter how to pack the correct foods for consumption during the final, crucial two or three days before stepping onstage.

There are many pitfalls to eating in restaurants. "Even a salad bar can get you into trouble during a contest cycle," explains Chrissie Glass (Los Angeles Champion and Light-weight California Champion). "Many restaurants spray a solution containing sodium on salad greens in order to preserve their freshness and color, and even a little sodium on food can badly bloat your body with water.

"A few restaurants don't use sodium on salad greens, so you should ask the manager of each restaurant if they do use sodium. It's a lot better to do this during the off-season than it is when your stomach is thinking that your throat has been cut. Identify two or three eating establishments without sodium-laden salad bars in your neighborhood, then patronize them whenever you are following a strict diet."

As Chrissie explains, it's even difficult at many restaurants to be sure you are receiving a sugar-free diet soda when you order one. "Refined sugar can be deadly when you're on a contest diet," she says, "and it's especially easy to consume a lot of sugar calories when you're drinking them. A sugared cola doesn't taste significantly different than its dietetic counterpart. And it's not that difficult for a waitress to accidentally draw you the wrong soda.

"The best way to avoid drinking sucrose calories in a soda is to either buy your soda in a can that is clearly labeled, or drink either iced tea or coffee sweetened with aspartame. You might even wish to tote your own can of soda with you to a restaurant and poor it into one of their glasses with some ice. Serious bodybuilders prefer to be safe rather than sorry."

Rice, potatoes, and pasta are staples in any low-calorie precontest diet, but when restaurant-cooked they can be fraught with unwanted fats. "Many restaurant cooks brush baked potatoes with oil or butter to 'improve the flavor,'" Glass explains. "If you like to eat the skins with your potatoes, the fats added to them can significantly increase the food's caloric value. Avoiding the potato skins can help, but sometimes the oil seeps through the skin into the meat of the potato. So, you should also question the restaurant manager about whether his potato skins have been brushed with butter or oil."

Sue Ann McKean (California Champion and a leading pro bodybuilder) warns about the dangers of eating restaurant rice and pasta. "No restaurant cook wants rice or pasta sticking to his cooking utensils, so he will frequently add butter or oil to the water in which he boils these foods. And each teaspoon of butter or oil which soaks into the rice or pasta increases the food's caloric content by approximately 100 calories.

"Since a gram of fat has more than twice as many calories in it than a gram of either protein or carbohydrate, you can most efficiently decrease your consumption of calories by cutting fats to a minimum. Rice and pasta provide plenty of bulk without being sources of concentrated calories, so you at least

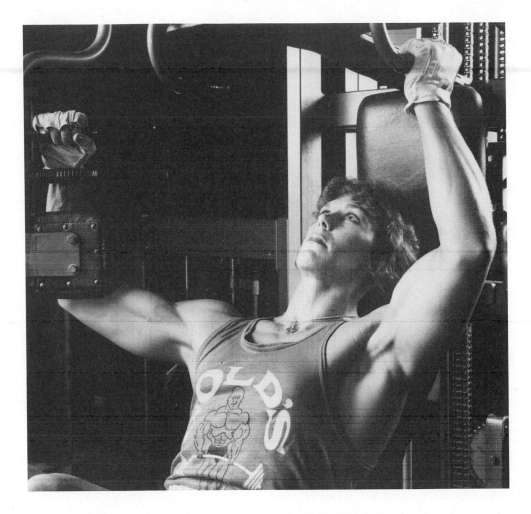

partially defeat the entire purpose of a low-calorie precontest diet when you eat rice or pasta that has been cooked in water with butter or oil—or even salt—added to it." Again, you must ask restaurant managers whether their cooks add anything to their cooking water.

"The chicken and tuna salads served in restaurants often contain hidden calories," adds Lee Labrada (National and World Middleweight Champion). "When my wife makes me tuna salad or chicken salad at home, she uses a bare minimum of a special low-calorie mayonnaise that she buys at a health food store. This way I can eat a tasty tuna salad or scrumptious chicken salad containing a low number of calories.

"Chicken and tuna salads found in restaurants are, by comparison, loaded with calories. Great gobs of regular, high-calorie mayo are used on restaurant salads, usually to the point where more than half of the calories in such salads come from the mayonnaise itself. But the extra calories don't stop with just the mayo, because restaurants also are cost-conscious. So, instead of using the lower calorie, higher costing albacore white tuna, they use less expensive dark tuna meat that has usually been packed in oil. They also use the darker meat from chicken legs instead of the white breast meat, and dark chicken meat is higher in calories.

"Chicken and tuna salad keep well in the fridge, and they make a taste-pleasing, bodybuilding snack, so you should have some on hand if you tend to be tempted by less healthy foods. Some supermarkets and virtually all health food stores sell a variety of low- and reduced-calorie mayonnaises. Always purchase this type of mayo rather than one with a great number of calories for use on your chicken salad and tuna salad.

"The chicken breasts used in chicken salad should be lightly broiled with the fatty skin removed before cooking. Water-packed chunk white tuna should be drained and rinsed in distilled water prior to use in a salad. Once you have the chicken cubed and the tuna broken up, use only enough low-cal mayo to coat the meat. Tuna or chicken salad prepared in this manner is a little more bland tasting than what you'd be likely to find in a restaurant, but it will do far more for you as a serious bodybuilder."

Chris Glass concludes, "If you can eat fresh fruit during a contest phase, avoid fruit cocktails and fruit salad at restaurants. Plain fruit doesn't stimulate the average person's palate. It isn't sweet enough for most diners, so restaurants often sprinkle refined sugar on their cut up fruit. It's better to eat a piece of whole fruit from a restaurant's salad bar."

So, what can a bodybuilder peaking for a show possibly eat at a restaurant? When eating out, a bodybuilder's best friend is a restaurant with a charcoal broiler, no sodium on the salad greens, and no oil or butter added to the baked potatoes, rice, and pasta.

Seafood can be broiled over an open fire with no oil or butter brushed on it, with rice, a salad with lemon juice squeezed over it, and an iced tea to provide a meal safe even for a bodybuilder a week out from a show. Or, you can eat a skinned and broiled chicken breast with a baked potato, salad, and coffee.

All of this may seem to be nit-picking to novice bodybuilders, but they will soon learn that they *must* pay attention to such small details if they hope to compete successfully at a high level. Bodybuilders who are careful of what they eat are usually successful bodybuilders.

PACKING FOR A COMPETITION

If you *do* want to be in perfect shape for an out-of-town show, it's essential for you to carry all of your own food and water to the competition. Failing to pack your own food will leave you at the mercy of unfamiliar restaurants when your mind should be focused only on your upcoming competition.

The next two chapters of this book will drive home how vital it is to consume the correct type of carbohydrates and totally avoid sodium right before a competition. And the *only* way to be sure you eat and drink correctly is to carry your own food and water to the show.

It's easy to eat correctly if you call ahead to be sure your hotel room has a refrigerator in it. A refrigerator costs an extra $5-$10 per day, but it's a good investment in your onstage appearance.

According to Chris Glass, "The best foods to carry with you to a show are amino acid capsules, the whites of hardboiled eggs, no-sodium rice cakes, boiled rice, baked potatoes, high-quality granola with no sugar added, and unsulfured dry fruit. You can carry either distilled water or Perrier water, which is sodium free. Eggs, potatoes, and rice keep well in a refrigerator and will stay fresh for up to three days even without cold storage."

Samir Bannout (Mr. Universe, Mr. World, Mr. Olympia) is one of the best organized bodybuilders prior to a competition. In a bag used just to pack food, he keeps every serving he will require, each one wrapped in tin foil and labeled with the precise date and time it is to be eaten. It's little wonder Samir has been so successful!

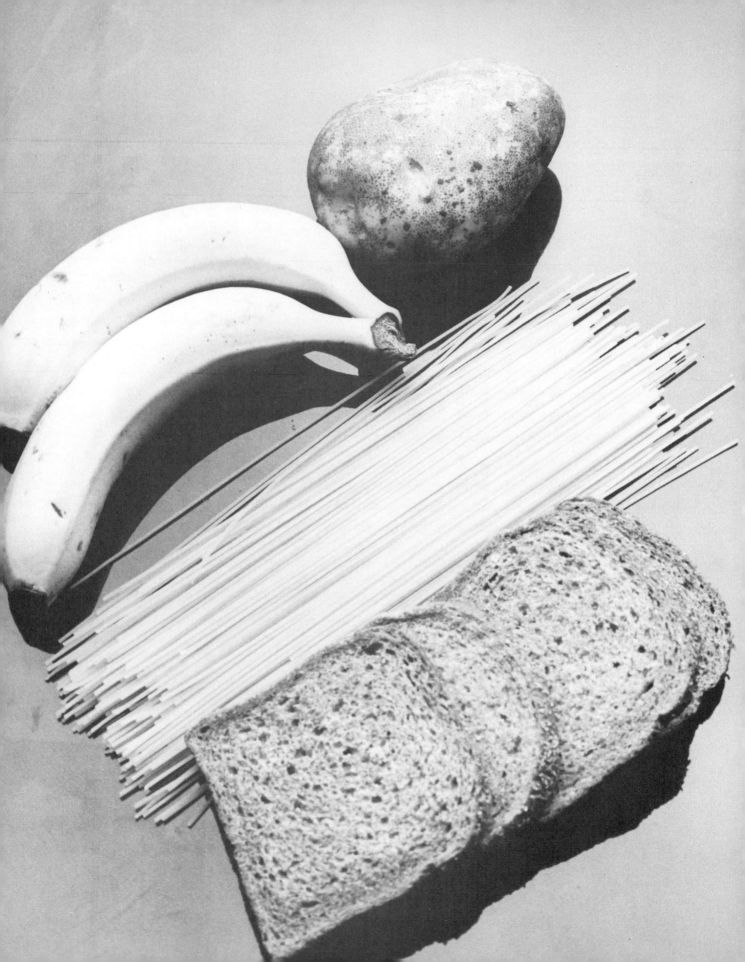

13
CARBOHYDRATE LOADING

As mentioned in Chapter 4, carbohydrate foods are your body's primary choice to provide fuel for the hard anaerobic training of a high-intensity bodybuilding workout. That's one reason why you will have so little training energy when you follow the low-carbohydrate precontest diet outlined in Chapter 11.

In order to fuel heavy mass-building sessions with the weights, you must be careful to consume a combination of complex and simple carbohydrate foods correctly timed at precise intervals between training sessions. Generally speaking, this is no problem during an off-season, mass-building training and dietary cycle because bodybuilders tend to eat excessive amounts of both complex and simple carbohydrates, and particularly excessive amounts of simple carbs. However, when you are dieting, you must take care to consume the right carbs at the correct time of day in order to ensure maximum-intensity workouts.

There is also a method recently in vogue in which a body-builder deprives his or her body of carbohydrates for a period of three to six days, during which the body becomes exhausted of stored carbohydrates. This deprivation phase is then followed by two to three days of carbohydrate loading in which plenty of complex carb foods are consumed. The combination of carbohydrate deprivation and loading pulls water from beneath the skin and from within the viscera and into the muscles and vascular system, making the muscles appear more full than ever before and the veins most prominent. This system of carbohydrate loading for a competition will be explained in detail near the end of this chapter.

WORKOUT CARB CONSUMPTION ON LOW-CARB DIETS

Have you ever attempted to follow a strict low-carbohydrate diet (less than 40–50 grams of carb foods per day) for an extended period of time? If you do, you will invariably discover that you completely run out of energy, both for workouts and everyday tasks, about the fourth or fifth day after commencing the diet. When you are training normally hard and doing about 30 minutes of aerobics per day, your physical energy expenditures will completely deplete glycogen (carbohydrate) from your muscles, liver, and vascular system within four to five days.

Once you hit energy rock bottom on a low-carb diet you should solve the problem by having one large meal high in complex carbohydrates like spaghetti and other pasta, potatoes, sweet potatoes, beans, legumes, and rice. This carb-loading meal should be eaten at night, and the meal will quickly restore you to normal—both in terms of physical energy and psychological mood—for another three to four days, at which point the high-carb meal should be repeated. And despite having one high-carb meal every three to five days when following a low-carb diet, you will notice that your muscularity gradually improves as body fat stores are mobilized to provide for daily energy needs on the zero- to low-carb meal days.

Virtually all champion bodybuilders—men and women alike—who adhere to low-carb diets eat at least one high-carb meal every three to five days without deleterious effect on reaching peak muscularity for a competition. And when they eat occasional meals high in complex carbohydrates, training energy is at a much higher level than on a strict low-carb precontest diet. In the end they retain much more ripped-up

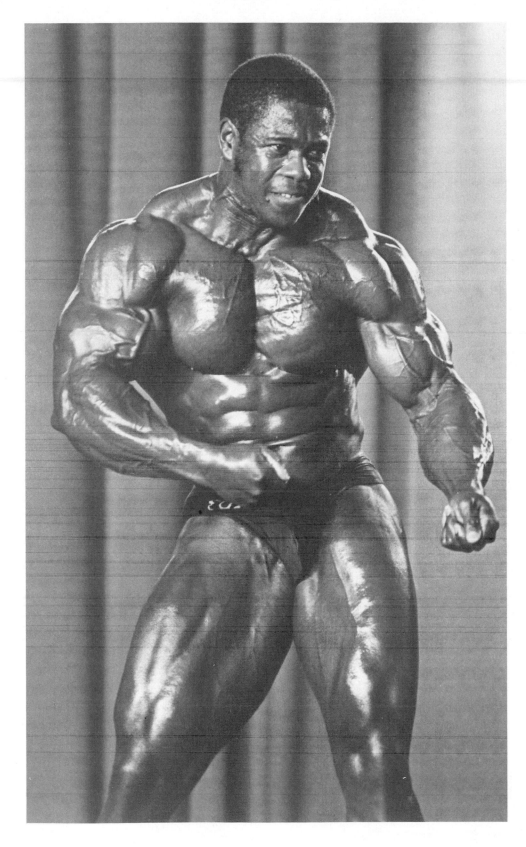

muscle mass onstage when they consume planned high-carb meals. And that's what bodybuilding is all about, isn't it? You want to go onstage with thick muscles, classic symmetry, perfect proportions, and optimum muscle density and muscularity. That's a winning combination.

WORKOUT CARB CONSUMPTION ON LOW-CALORIE DIETS

When you're following a low-fat/low-calorie diet prior to an important competition, you'll be able to pretty much consume any natural carb foods you might like. But the choice and timing of carbohydrate food consumption is a critical factor in augmenting energy levels.

Primarily, you should eat complex carbohydrate foods year-round, including during the contest preparatory phase. But you should limit your consumption of simple carbs from fruit and other sources during an off-season cycle because they tend to cause an excessively extreme energy spike soon after you have eaten the food.

Depending on the time of day at which you wish to train, you should eat some type of complex carbohydrate food—a baked potato or two, a bowl of rice, some whole grains—at least two hours before your training session. This will give you plenty of slow carbohydrate energy because complex carbohydrate foods break down more slowly in your digestive system and provide sustained energy over a longer period of time than do simple carbs.

About 45–60 minutes before training, you can consume a serving or two of simple carbohydrate foods. Let's let Gold's Gym member, Tom Platz (Mr. Universe) tell you about his preworkout meal: "I generally consume two bananas, two Pop Tarts, a glass of juice, and a cup of coffee to get my blood circulating. Some people might object to the Pop Tarts, but they probably haven't read the nutrition breakdown on this little delicacy. Two Pop Tarts contain 400 calories, 80 grams of carbohydrates—consisting of starches and quick sugars—and only eight grams of fat. For me this is the perfect precontest meal, and I can blast my muscles to the limit for two to three straight hours without losing any energy momentum."

CARB LOADING FOR COMPETITION

Chris Glass (Los Angeles Champion, California Lightweight Champion) gave the best account of carbohydrate loading that we have seen in one of her *Flex* magazine articles. She wrote, "You'll want to vary the carbo deprivation/loading if you are attempting to make a weight class. But when optimally carried out, this technique allows you to divert definition-blurring water from beneath your skin to your muscles. As a result, you look more massive and cut up. However you need a very strong mind in order to correctly carry out the process.

"Here is my basic program: Six days before competing, I cut my carbohydrate consumption from its usual precontest level of 100–120 grams per day (the minimum amount I need to provide workout energy and aid full recovery between workouts) to 50 grams or fewer. Combined with plenty of anaerobic and aerobic exercise, this depletes my muscles, liver, and vascular system of glycogen. As a result, I appear so flat and small the final deprivation day that I'm always tempted to drop out of the show. But by sticking it out, I end up looking better than ever onstage.

"The last two days prior to competing, I carb load by consuming 130–150 grams per day of complex carbohydrate foods only, such as rice and potatoes. And the morning of the show I eat small quantities of dried fruit to increase energy for the prejudging without filling out my stomach and enlarging my waistline. I also keep my liquid consumption down to the point where I am a little thirsty at all times.

"When the body is deprived of carbohydrates and then fed with carbs, it responds by storing a greater-than-normal amount of glycogen in the muscles, liver, and vascular system. Glycogen attracts approximately four times its weight in water, sucking fluid away from the skin and into the muscles and bloodstream, causing you to appear more massive, ripped, and vascular than you would if you hadn't manipulated your carbohydrate consumption.

"Four days of carbohydrate depletion is perfect for my body, though you may need to add or subtract a day to your regimen. But keep this fact in mind: the longer you deplete your body of

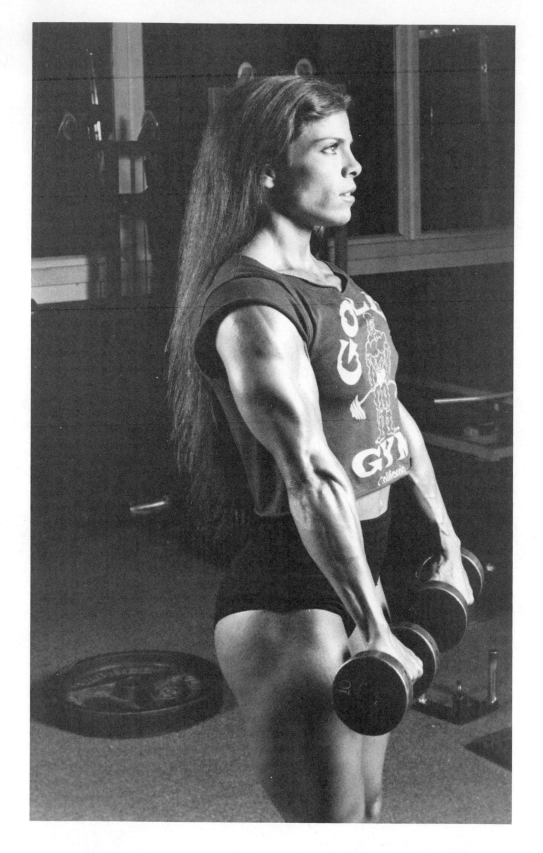

carbohydrates, the better your chances are of losing muscle mass. Therefore, it would be a good idea to have a dry run or two of carbohydrate manipulation several weeks or months before your show in order to determine how many depletion and loading days work best for you."

When you are carb depleting/loading and sodium loading/depleting, your body will look absolutely terrible three to four days out from the show. "But that's when you have to have a strong mind," notes Scott Wilson (Mr. California, Mr. International). "There's no doubt that both of these processes work well to bring your body to a perfect peak for a competition, but when you are looking small from depleting carbohydrates and looking smooth as a baby's behind from consuming so much salt, it takes great mental discipline to continue with the program.

"I've known plenty of young men and women who have made the mistake of dropping out of a show, only to discover that they look fantastic on the day of the competition. Be strong mentally, and this won't happen to you. You'll look like a champion, and bring home a first-place trophy!"

Virtually all of the Gold's Gym champions manipulate carbohydrate intake prior to a competition, but a few don't, and they have also been very successful in entering competitions with optimum muscle mass and muscularity. So, you should experiment with both carbohydrate depletion/loading and with merely entering a competition while eating normally and monitoring sodium intake so that you don't appear bloated with water onstage.

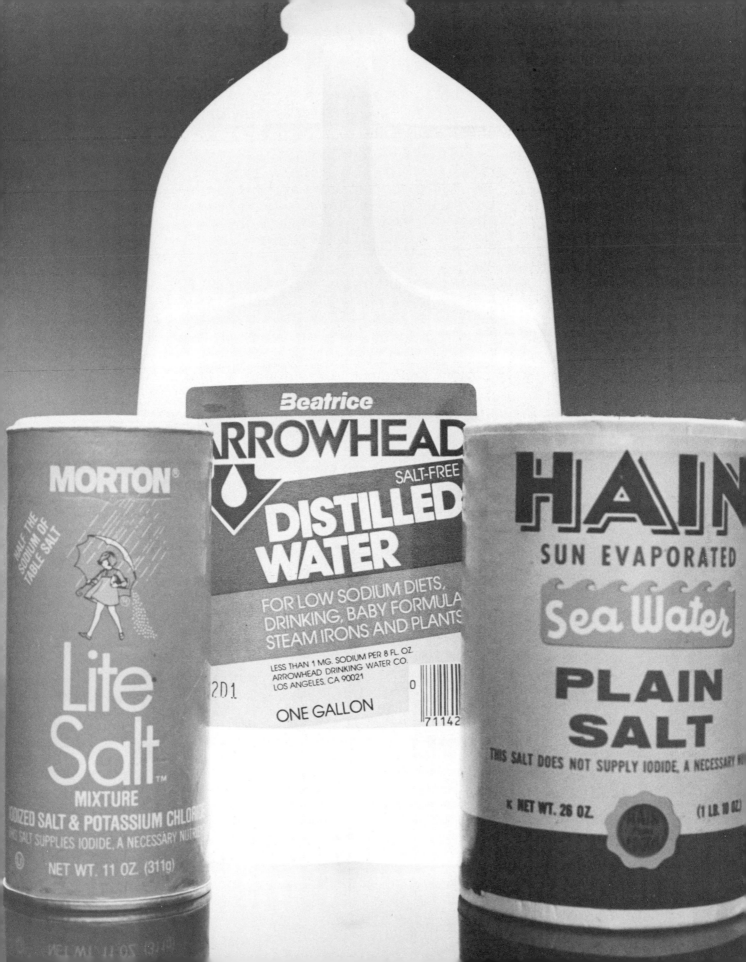

14
BODY WATER BALANCE

"On the day of a competition," notes Lee Labrada (National and World Champion), "it's absolutely essential that you have a maximum amount of water in your muscles and vascular system, and the minimum possible amount of water anywhere else in your body. Nothing, for example, can kill your chances at a competition faster than walking onstage with plenty of muscle mass distributed symmetrically and proportionately on your body, but with your paper-thin skin bloated with water sufficiently to make you appear smooth at a prejudging."

There are several factors that have a direct bearing on the distribution of water within your body. In the previous chapter, you learned how first depriving your system of carbohydrates for several days and then loading up with carbs will attract nearly all of the water beneath your skin and move it into your muscles and vascular system, giving you a big, ripped-up appearance for your competition.

The amount of sodium in your body can also have a direct bearing on body water retention. The secretion of a hormone called aldosterone, which is produced in much greater than normal quantities when a bodybuilder is under the stress of an upcoming competition, can cause considerable water retention. Allergies to certain foods—most notably grains and milk prod-

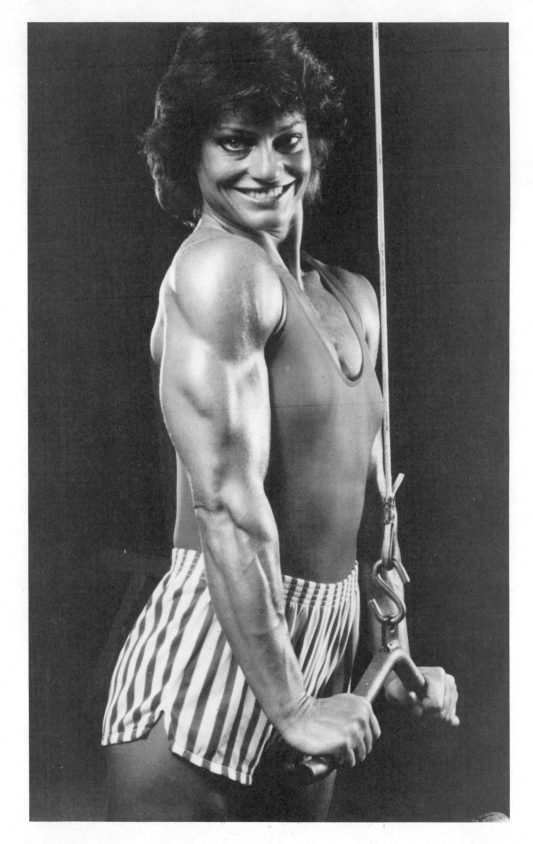

ucts—can retain excess water in your body, too. And women bodybuilders at certain phases of their menstrual cycles will retain more water than normal.

DIURETICS

Diuretics are drugs that stimulate urination and thereby dehydrate your body. Many bodybuilders, notably those in Europe, rely heavily on diuretics to give their bodies a very hard appearance for a competition. But harsh chemical diuretics can be very dangerous because they leach from your body chemicals necessary for proper function of the heart. There are two substantiated reports of European bodybuilders, one a former IFBB World Champion and the other a Swedish Junior competitor, who have taken excessive dosages of diuretics and died in the process.

High percentages of competitive bodybuilders use diuretics in order to maximize muscularity for a competition. Usually, this is done when a bodybuilder has come up a bit short in his or her diet and fears appearing smooth onstage. The use of harsh chemical diuretics does reduce the amount of water in an athlete's body, giving the illusion of greater muscularity. But diuretics can also cause serious cramps in major muscle groups, and they definitely cause a diminishment of muscle mass.

Muscles are made up of more than 70 percent water, and when you remove water from your muscles with a diuretic, they appear to be smaller. When it's relatively easy to diet down to the point where you have no visible body fat and can still display large muscles, it makes little sense to mistime your diet, come up a little fat, and then injure your body by using harsh diuretics.

If you are a woman and holding water due to your menstrual cycle, you might benefit from the use of mild herbal diuretic. There are several brands of these at health food stores.

While we certainly don't recommend this practice, many male and female bodybuilders take heavy dosages of laxatives the night before a competition. These athletes report that the laxatives remove water from the body, and primarily from the upper thighs, hips, buttocks, and abdomen. And after an augmented morning bowel movement, an athlete's abdomen will be flat, and the abdominal muscles will be much easier to contract. Again, we don't recommend the use of laxatives prior to a competition, but if you do, you should experiment with various brands and dosage levels at some time prior to your competition in order to determine which formula works best for you.

SODIUM

Sodium is one of the four main electrolyte minerals responsible for proper nerve function and strong, sustained muscle contractions. The other three electrolytes are calcium, magnesium, and potassium. The AMDR for sodium is quite low, however, only 200 milligrams per day. Even a hard-training bodybuilder who perspires freely for two or three hours per day needs no more than 400–500 milligrams of sodium.

Since sodium has such a high affinity for water, it retains more than 50 times its weight in water in your body. That's why most bodybuilders severely limit sodium consumption for days or even weeks prior to a competition. It's unwise, however, to limit sodium for more than two to three days prior to a show because your body will react much more dramatically to sodium consumption when it has been deprived of the mineral.

The simplest way to achieve a proper water balance onstage is to consume 300–400 milligrams of sodium per day for three weeks up to the final week prior to competing. Then sodium intake should be cut to 50 milligrams or less for the final week, and as close as possible to zero for the final two to three days prior to competing.

SODIUM LOADING

A new process of sodium loading and deprivation has been used since the mid–1980s to bring bodybuilders onstage in perfect shape and with absolutely no excess water retention. This process is used by virtually every top champ, and you can experiment with it during an off-season cycle to determine how much sodium you should consume when loading, how long you should sodium load, and how long you should avoid sodium before your competition.

Stress and sodium deprivation can both be causes of aldosterone secretion, which in turn will cause unwanted water

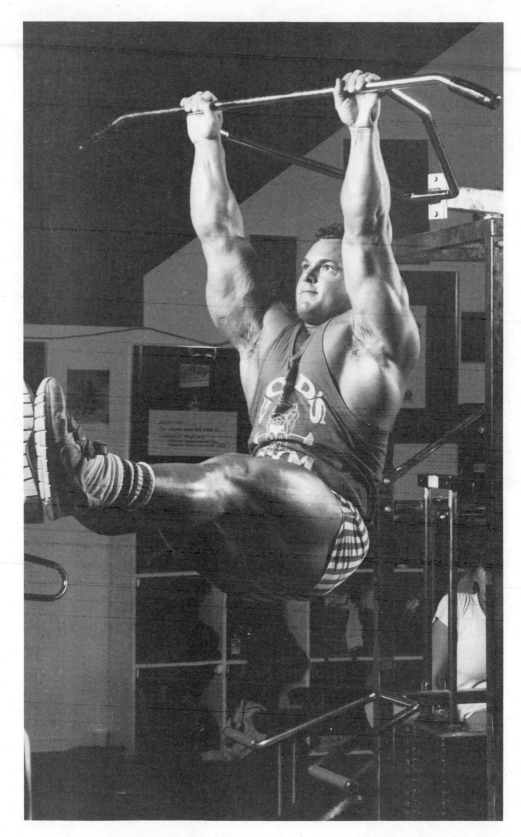

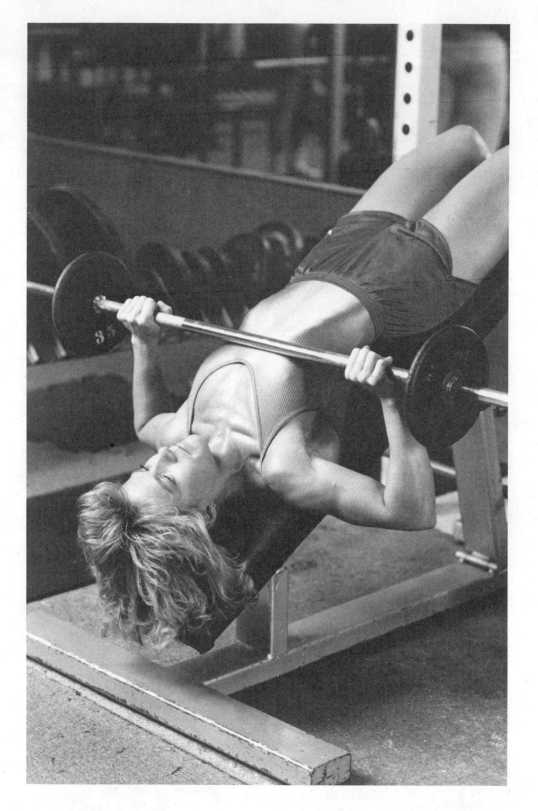

retention. But by correctly sodium loading and then sodium depleting, you can fake out your body and keep it from secreting aldosterone. This process takes a total of seven to eight days. For the first four to five days, you will consume excess quantities of sodium, gradually working up from one gram per day to three or four grams the final sodium-loading day. This large sodium intake keeps your body from secreting any aldosterone. And it's also important to know that your body is slow to secrete aldosterone once you cut sodium from your diet completely. It takes three to four days for your body to begin aldosterone secretion.

After loading up on sodium for four to five days, you must then cut your dietary sodium intake to zero or as close to zero as possible. This even means eating fresh-water fish rather than salt-water fish. For the first couple of days, you'll look like the dog's dinner, bloated with water. But since sodium passes through your body in 48–72 hours, you will soon find yourself ripping up like never before. And on the actual day of your competition, you will have no sodium in your body to hold water and blur out your contest-winning cuts.

THE ALDOSTERONE PROBLEM

Everyone is nervous when a competition is approaching, but some bodybuilders are so hyper that the stress of the upcoming show causes their bodies to secret aldosterone even when a sodium loading-deprivation cycle has been followed to the letter. We can recall one famous bodybuilder who always looked great a couple of days before the show, was waterlogged to the gills onstage, and then looked ripped to rags again a day or two after the show. Ultimately, it was established that his problem was aldosterone secretion caused by the stress he was under due to his excitable personality.

At times, aldosterone problems can be solved by practicing relaxation techniques. But the easiest way to combat aldosterone is to ask your family physician for an Aldactone prescription. Aldactone counteracts aldosterone quite effectively. But please keep in mind that we do not presume to prescribe drugs in this book. You should carefully discuss all potential side effects of Aldactone with your physician before deciding to use it.

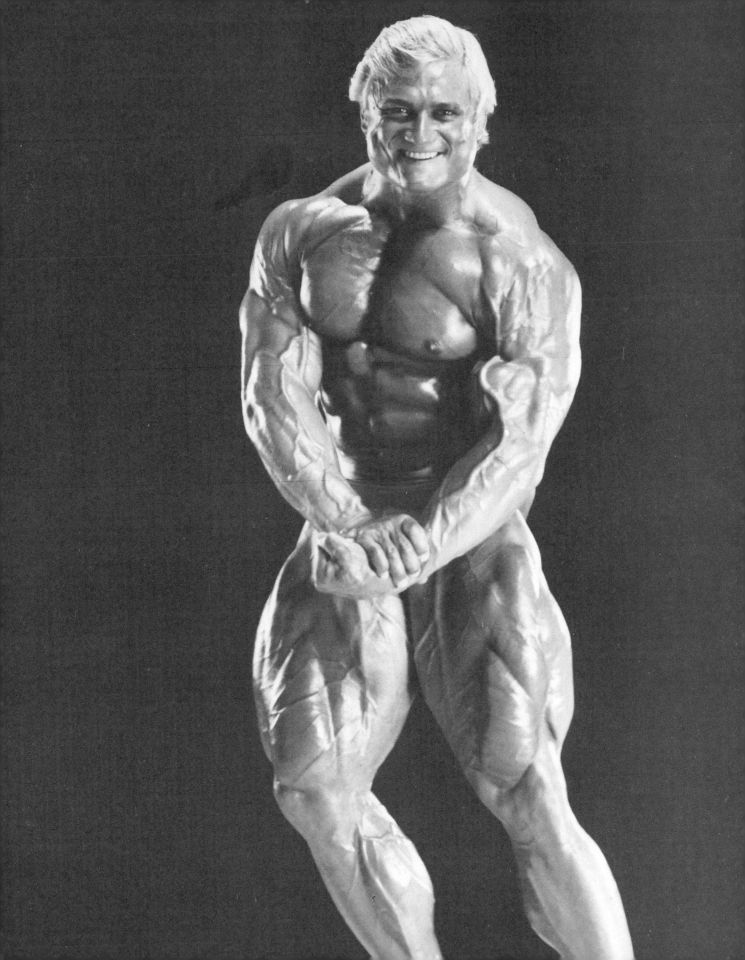

15
THE CYCLE TRAINING
AND DIETING PRINCIPLE

One of the biggest secrets of developing the extreme muscle mass and sharp muscularity of today's crop of superstar bodybuilders has been the cycling of off-season training and diet to build up muscle mass with cycles of precontest training and diet intended to refine the mass built up in the off-season. Virtually all top male and female bodybuilders of the current era follow this cycling principle.

Chapter 9 outlined training and dietary strategies for building up muscle mass, and these are the precise strategies that you will use during an off-season preparatory cycle. In order to synthesize the entire off-season and precontest cycles, I'll repeat much of what I discussed in Chapter 9, as well as much of the information in Chapter 11, which thoroughly discussed precontest diet.

OFF-SEASON TRAINING

You should have two primary objectives when embarking on an off-season training cycle. The first is to add to general body muscle mass, and the second is to particularly improve a weak body part or two that has been holding you back from winning the big titles. And the efficiency with which you improve weak points and generally increase muscle mass will make or break you as a competitive bodybuilder.

Each time you peak for a competition, you should have as many photos as possible taken of your physique so that you can evaluate its strong and weak points. Ed Corney (Mr. America, Mr. Universe) said, "When I was competing, even past the age of 50, I was always overjoyed to receive snapshots from my fans. Even if these photos were taken from poor angles, I was always able to learn something from a picture. I'd see that the inner heads of my calves or the posterior heads of my deltoids needed additional work, and by the time I competed again, I would have them up to par with the remainder of my physique."

Tom Platz (Mr. Universe) is another bodybuilder who loves to receive photos from his legion of fans: "I particularly like to get photos that I don't like, because they're the ones which most vividly display the weaknesses in my physique. For the longest time, my upper body lagged far behind my legs, and I could clearly see this in the photos that fans sent me. I'd put those pictures that showed me at my worst on my bathroom mirror so I'd be forced to see them every day. And in turn this kindled a burning desire to improve my weak areas, which I was able to do and win the IFBB Mr. Universe title in Acapulco, Mexico, and later place second in the Pro Mr. Universe and third in the Mr. Olympia competitions."

Self-evaluations can be made by pouring over the myriad photos an experienced photographer has taken of you a few days before or after your competition. One such case occurred in the late 1960s when entrepreneur Joe Weider sponsored the soon-to-be-great Arnold Schwarzenegger over to the United States from West Germany to train in southern California. After sifting through all of his photos, the Austrian Oak decided that his calves were his weak point.

So that he could be constantly aware of how bad his calves were, Arnold carefully cut off the legs of all of his sweat pants just above the knees. This way, he was constantly reminded of his calf weakness, which induced him to train them with much greater intensity than at any other time in the past. Taking a hint from his hero at the time, Reg Park (four times Mr. Universe), Arnold began doing sets of super-heavy Standing Calf Raises every other day, and soon his calves were among the best in the sport, harmonizing beautifully with what many bodybuilding aficionados consider the greatest physique to ever step onstage for a competition.

Only a minority of bodybuilders are able to look in the mirror and objectively evaluate their physical development. It's usually much easier to arrive at an objective evaluation of your physique if you spend hours pouring over your latest photos. But even then, you may miss a key weakness or two, which will spell disaster when you step onstage.

For the most part, it's best to have an acknowledged expert such as Bill Pearl (Mr. America, Mr. USA, four times Mr. Universe) evaluate your physique in person. Unless you live in the back woods and train in your garage, you will be able to find a top bodybuilder or experienced gym owner who will be only too happy to give you an objective evaluation from time to time on what you most need to work in order to bring your physical proportions into perfect balance. I wouldn't, however, suggest that you ask one of your main competitors for an evaluation because he or she might not be totally honest, seeing a chance to lead you astray and induce you to further overdevelop an already strong body part.

As long as you are tactful and polite, one of the best ways of identifying weak points in your physique—as well as in your general stage presence and posing—is to approach two or three judges after each competition. Maintain an attitude of wanting to learn and constantly improve yourself, and judges will go out of their way to help you. But if you are belligerent, forget it. We've seen too many young bodybuilders told that their calves were underpar, only to scream, "My calves are great! Just look at them!" And he rolls up his pants to display a couple of Popsicle sticks. No judge will ever waste time on such a bodybuilder, and the same judges seem to crop up at virtually every competition.

Once you have identified a weak area or two, you must formulate an attack to bring those lagging areas up. Actually, it's much easier to bring up one body part, but you can usually bring up two muscle groups as long as one of them is relatively small, such as a triceps weakness. But if you're trying to simultaneously bring up your thigh and back muscles, which are the largest in your body, you will be doomed to failure.

You should use the Muscle Priority System on a weak body part. This system involves training the weak body part first in your routine when you have maximum stores of mental and physical energy to devote to bombing the laggard to the max.

Let's say that you are a fairly experienced bodybuilder who has lagging deltoids. Following a four-day split routine accenting shoulder development, you might train like this:

MONDAY–THURSDAY

Exercise	Sets	Reps
Hanging Leg Raises	3	15–20
Roman Chair Sit-Ups	3	20–30
Cable Upright Rows	5	15–6*
Seated Presses Behind Neck	5	15–6*
Dumbbell Bent Laterals	3–4	8–10
One-Arm Cable Side Laterals	3–4	8–10
Standing Barbell Curls	4	8–10
Cable Preacher Curls	4	8–10
Close-Grip Bench Presses	4	8–10
Pulley Pushdowns	4	8–10
Barbell Reverse Curls	4	8–10
Barbell Wrist Curls	4	15–20
Standing Calf Raises	4–5	10–15
Donkey Calf Raises	4–5	15–20

Note: Exercises marked with an asterisk are performed as a half pyramid, the weights increased each set as the reps are progressively lowered. In this case, you can do 15, 12, 10, 8, and 6 reps in your five sets each of Cable Upright Rows and Seated Presses Behind Neck.

TUESDAY–FRIDAY

Exercise	Sets	Reps
Incline Sit-Ups	3	20–25
Bench Leg Raises	3	25–30
Hyperextensions	3	15–20
Squats	5	15–6*
Leg Curls	4	10–12
Seated Pulley Rows	5	15–6*
Barbell Shrugs	4	10–15
Barbell Bench Presses	5	15–6*
Incline Dumbbell Presses	4	8–10
Parallel Bar Dips	3–4	maximum
Cross-Bench Dumbbell Pullovers	2–3	10–15
Seated Calf Raises	5	8–10

Note: Exercises marked with an asterisk are performed as a half pyramid, the weights increased each set as the reps are progressively lowered.

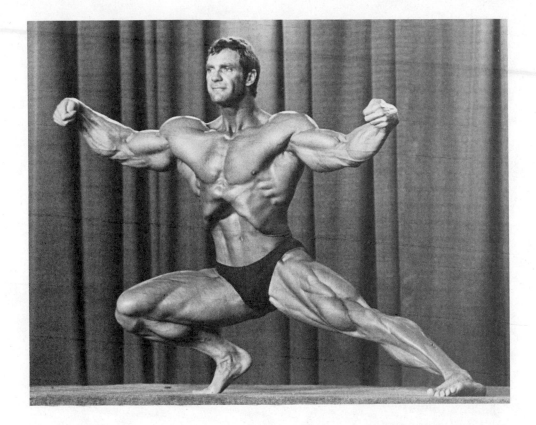

When arms and legs are particularly weak points, they should be priority-trained by themselves twice a week, with the remainder of your body trained the other two days. Following is the way massive Lou Ferrigno brought up his legs and began to win national and later international titles:

MONDAY–THURSDAY

Exercise	Sets	Reps
Roman Chair Sit-Ups	3–4	25–30
Seated Twisting	3–4	50–100
Leg Extensions (light, as a warm-up)	4	15–20
Squats	10	20–2*
Leg Presses	5	15–6*
Hack Squats	5	15–6*
Lying Leg Curls	4	12–6*
Standing Leg Curls	4	12–6*
Stiff-Legged Deadlifts	4	10–15
Seated Calf Raises	5	8–12
Standing Calf Raises	5	15–20
Calf Presses	5	20–30

Note: Squats were done as a half pyramid using reps of 20, 18, 16, 14, 12, 10, 8, 6, 4, and 2, increasing the poundage with each succeeding set until he was using absolute maximum weights for the last three to four sets. Leg Presses and Hack Squats were done with reps of 15, 12, 10, 8, and 6 with the weight increased after each set. And Lying Leg Curls and Standing Leg Curls were performed for reps of 12, 10, 8, and 6 with the weight increased after each set until the last one to two sets were performed at limit intensity.

TUESDAY–FRIDAY

Exercise	Sets	Reps
Hanging Leg Raises	3	10–15
Incline Sit-Ups	3	20–30
Incline Barbell Presses	6	15–4*
Barbell Bench Press to Neck	4	10–12
Parallel Bar Dips (weighted)	4	8–12
Machine Presses Behind Neck	6	15–4*
Barbell Upright Rows	4	12–6*
Seated Dumbbell Side Laterals	4	8–12
Dumbbell Bent Laterals	4	8–12
Chins	4	10–12
Barbell Bent Rows (standing on bench)	4	8–12
Seated Pulley Rows	4	8–12
Seated Dumbbell Curls	4	8–12
Barbell Preacher Curls	4	8–12
Lying Barbell Triceps Extensions	4	8–12
Lat Pushdowns	4	8–12
Barbell Reverse Curls	4	8–12
One-Arm Dumbbell Wrist Curls	4	8–12

Note: Pyramid sets and reps of exercises marked with an asterisk.

When your arms are a weak point, you must train them separately from the remainder of your torso muscle groups, because your biceps and triceps come into play so strongly in chest, back, and shoulder movements. If you trained arms first and then attempted to do your torso exercises, you would not be able to receive much benefit from the torso exercises.

Following is a sample muscle priority training program for use in bringing up lagging arm muscles:

MONDAY–THURSDAY

Exercise	Sets	Reps
Incline Leg Raises	3	20–30
Twisting Incline Sit-Ups	3	20–30
Wide-Grip Standing Barbell Curls	4	8–10
Incline Dumbbell Curls	4	8–10
Cable Preacher Curls (bar handle)	4	8–10
Standing Dumbbell Concentration Curls	4	8–10
Triceps Parallel Bar Dips (torso erect)	4	8–10
Standing Two-Arm Dumbbell Triceps Extensions	4	8–10
Lying Barbell Triceps Extensions	4	8–10
Dumbbell Kickbacks	4	8–10
Barbell Reverse Curls	4	8–10
Barbell Reverse Wrist Curls	4	8–10
Standing Calf Raises	5	8–10
Calf Presses	5	15–20
Neck Strap Movement	4	10–15

TUESDAY–FRIDAY

Exercise	Sets	Reps
Hanging Leg Raises	3	10–15
Roman Chair Sit-Ups	3	25–30
Hyperextensions	3	15–20
Leg Extensions (warm-up only)	4	15–20
Squats	6	15–4*
Lying Leg Curls	4	10–15
Stiff-Legged Deadlifts	4	10–15
Seated Low Pulley Rows	4	8–10
Pulldowns Behind Neck	4	8–10
Nautilus Pullovers	4	10–15
Machine Front Presses	6	15–4*
Nautilus Side Laterals	4	10–12
Cable Bent Laterals	4	10–12
Machine Incline Presses	6	15–4*
Machine Decline Presses	4	12–6*
Pec Deck Flyes	4	8–10
Seated Calf Raises	5	8–12
One-Legged Dumbbell Calf Raises	5	15–20

Note: Pyramid weights and reps on all exercises marked with an asterisk.

In order to develop huge muscle mass, your objective during an off-season cycle must be to train as heavily as possible for relatively low reps (three to six on the heaviest sets) primarily on basic exercises such as Squats, Bench Presses, Seated Pulley Rows, Barbell Curls, Chins, Seated Pulley Rows, Deadlifts, and Parallel Bar Dips. And it is very important that you both warm up thoroughly on each major movement in your routine and use impeccable biomechanics (form) on every movement so that you obtain the greatest amount of stress from each set without risking injury.

A TRAINING TRANSITION CYCLE

Once you have completed a competition, you should take a two- to three-week layoff from training to heal up any minor injuries you might have incurred when training with maximum intensity for a competitive peak. A short layoff will also refresh your mind and make you desire to get back into the gym to start gearing up for another competition.

It is very injurious to your body to jump from a peaking cycle and peaking diet right into an off-season mass-building program and diet, and vice-versa. In order to keep from shocking your body unduly, you should take a two- or three-week transitional cycle between precontest and off-season cycles.

Following a post-competition layoff, you should start back into the gym with only three light workouts the first week, merely doing about five sets per body part to loosen up your joints and muscles. The second week, you can move up to doing a four-day split routine, increasing the intensity of your workout about 25 percent. Beginning with the third week, you can adopt the three-on-one-off training routine that you will use in the off-season, three training days followed by a day of rest. But you should not work out with maximum intensity until about the fourth or fifth week back in the gym. Without building up slowly like this, you would probably risk a minor injury or perhaps overtrain.

OFF-SEASON DIET

Your off-season diet was outlined in detail in Chapter 13, so I will only touch upon the high points here. As with the gradual transition in training intensity between precontest and off-season cycles, you must also cycle your diet up to a true off-season regimen. It's virtually impossible for any bodybuilder to avoid consuming massive quantities of cheesecake, ice cream, and other junk foods in the two or three weeks following a peak. But most men and women tend to burn out on the junk food after only a few weeks.

As soon as you begin to cycle up to an off-season training program, you should also cycle your diet up to an off-season regimen. This is accomplished by eliminating outright junk foods and gradually replacing them with high-quality complex carbohydrate foods such as potatoes, sweet potatoes, and rice. Consume plenty of salads, fresh veggies, white meats (poultry without the fatty skin and fish), eggs, limited milk products, grains, cereals, and heavy breads.

Following are the primary factors that should be considered when formulating an off-season diet:

1. Consume four to six smaller meals rich in protein rather than the two or three meals that most people enjoy.

2. Consume approximately one gram of high-quality protein per pound of body weight each day.

3. Use a powdered protein supplement mixed in milk with a banana or other soft fruit in a blender for use whenever you might be inclined to miss a meal.

4. If your budget allows you to purchase quality free-form amino acid capsules, use 10–15 of them throughout the day, but particularly 30 minutes before a workout and about halfway through each training session. Free-form amino acids are a very efficient source of dietary protein, as well as a means of increasing training energy and a sense of well-being.

5. Try to consume no more than 20 grams of protein foods or protein supplements each time you eat.

6. Consume primarily complex carbohydrate foods, such as potatoes, rice, legumes, beans, sweet potatoes, and vegetables.

7. If you need a quick energy boost just before a workout, eat the simple carbs found in one or two pieces of fruit.

8. Consume less protein during the evening than in the morning. Heavy protein meals at night can make you feel sluggish the next morning when you try to train. It's best to eat complex carbohydrates with a few free-form amino acid capsules at night.

9. Take one to two multipacks of vitamins, minerals and

trace elements with meals each day. You should also take supplemental vitamin C and vitamin B-complex each day in addition to the multipacks.

10. Avoid unnecessary junk food consumption. A scoop of ice cream or a good quality cookie now and then won't kill you, but don't make a habit of eating a quart of ice cream every night. It'll only make you as fat as a pig.

A DIETARY TRANSITION CYCLE

The point at which you begin to diet for a competition depends on how out of shape you are at that particular point and on how quickly you can lose the body fat that obscures your hard-earned muscles. Most experienced bodybuilders allow six to ten weeks in order to reach optimum condition. The first two to three weeks of dieting are devoted to a gradual break-in from the heavier eating of an off-season cycle to lighter precontest diet. Also, every successful bodybuilder gradually reduces the number of calories consumed each succeeding week because the body's metabolism tends to slow when it senses that it is being deprived of its normal amount of food.

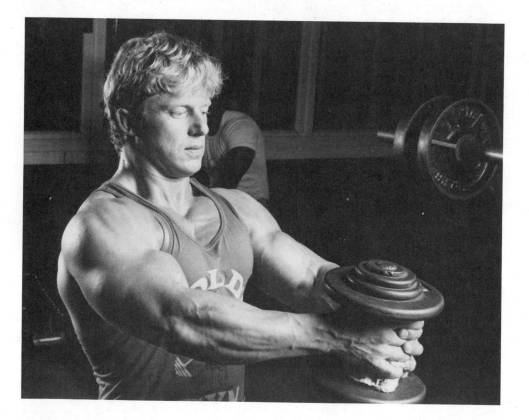

PRECONTEST DIET

The best precontest diet is healthily balanced, but low in fat content and hence low in calories. By consuming small amounts of chicken, turkey, and fish in addition to salads, potatoes, rice, and sweet potatoes, you will be able to gradually and effectively strip all excess fat from your body, revealing a championship physique.

You will also find that you will make your best progress in losing body fat if you consume four smaller meals each day rather than only two to three. This keeps your blood sugar up throughout the day, making it easy to do your weight workouts and aerobics sessions.

Following is a sample precontest, low-calorie diet you might use to harden up for a competition:

- *Meal 1*—poached egg whites, bran cereal with nonfat milk, multipack of supplements
- *Meal 2*—broiled chicken breast (skinned before cooking), rice, salad, iced tea with aspartame.
- *Meal 3*—tuna salad with minimum of dressing, slice of heavy bread, ice water, multipack of supplements
- *Meal 4*—broiled fish, dry baked potato, green vegetable, slice of watermelon, coffee

PRECONTEST TRAINING

Precontest training programs are as unique as all bodybuilders are unique. Some very successful bodybuilders use precisely the same routine year-round. Others simply train with the same degree of intensity while adding greatly to the number of sets they perform for each body part. And some merely increase the number of reps they perform of each movement without otherwise modifying the training program.

Still, most bodybuilders gradually cycle up to a precontest training program that is remarkably similar to those used by most other bodybuilders. To begin with, a bodybuilder begins to quality train, that is, to gradually reduce the length of rest intervals between sets from an average of 1½–2 minutes during the off-season to about 30–45 seconds between sets. Repetitions are also increased slightly, and most bodybuilders gradually do more total sets per muscle group.

During an off-season cycle, most of the sets you perform in

your routine should be basic exercises designed to pack on the most possible muscle mass in the shortest possible time. But as a competition approaches, an intelligent bodybuilder switches over to doing far more isolation movements than basic exercises. Still, at least one basic movement is included in the routine in an effort to maintain the greatest possible degree of muscle mass while training down and reaching competition shape.

Following are off-season and precontest training programs for the chest that you can use to determine the difference between these training modes:

OFF-SEASON

Exercise	Sets	Reps
Barbell Bench Press	6	15–6*
Incline Machine Presses	6	15–6*
Parallel Bar Dips (weighted)	6	10–15
Cross-Bench Pullovers	2–3	10–15

PRECONTEST

Exercise	Sets	Reps
Incline Machine Presses	6	15–6*
Pec Deck Flyes	4	10–12
Incline Dumbbell Flyes	4	10–12
Decline Cable Flyes	4	10–12
Cable Crossovers	4	10–12
Cross-Bench Pullovers	4	10–15

Note: Pyramid weights and reps on all exercises marked with an asterisk.

There are several training intensification techniques that you should also use in your quest to achieve peak muscle mass, density, and muscularity. One of these is forced reps, in which your training partner pulls up on the bar just enough to allow you to force out two to three reps past the point at which you should normally be forced to quit a set.

Peak contraction is also used quite frequently. With this technique, you choose movements (e.g., leg extensions) in which you have a maximum weight on the working muscles when they are in a fully contracted position. Holding the peak contracted position for a slow count of one or two gives your quadriceps striations like nothing else can.

You should also use continuous tension in your workouts. This technique involves moving the weights slowly along the full range of motion for each exercise, feeling the weight every inch of the way. You will find it best to powerfully contract both the working muscles and the antagonistic muscles for each of the muscles that are being worked. And be sure to slowly move the weights over the full range of motion of each exercise.

Finally, you should use iso-tension contraction exercises without weights each day for the final weeks leading up to your competition. Iso-tension consists of very powerful flexes of each muscle group, the flexes lasting six to eight seconds. Rest intervals of about 10 seconds are taken between rep flexes, and as many as 50 reps are performed for each muscle group.

If you've done your training and dietary homework efficiently, you should be in peak condition on the day of your competition. After the euporia has worn off and the trophy is on your mantelpiece, take another two- or three-week layoff from hard training and then gradually work up in intensity for another important competition.

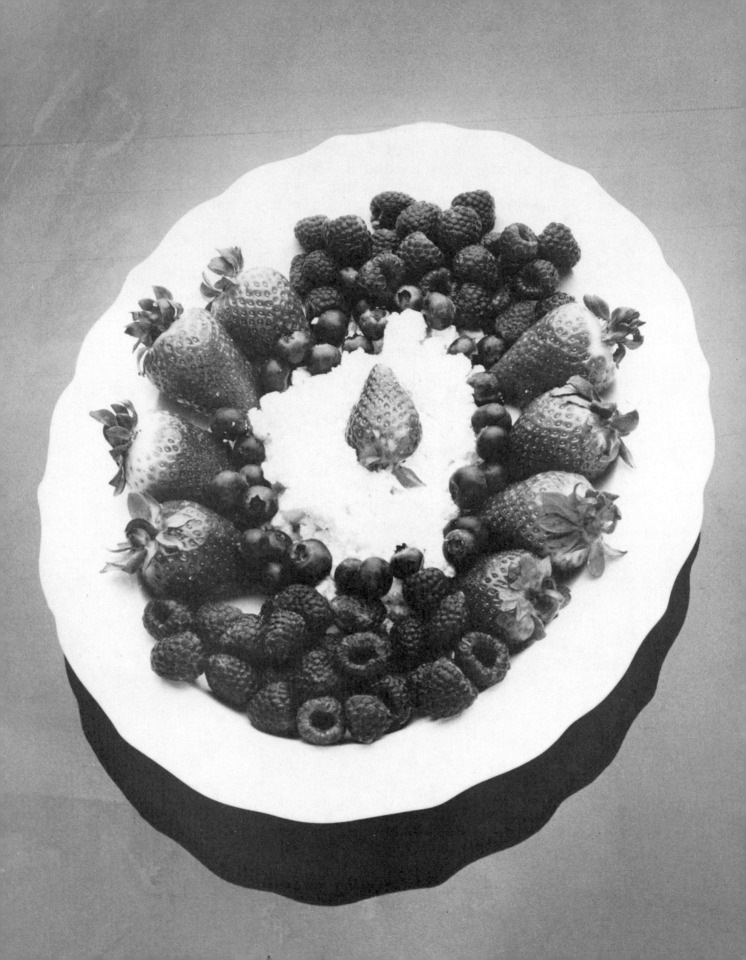

16
HOW TO NUTRITIONALLY INCREASE TRAINING ENERGY

An excess of energy is invaluable to any serious, hardtraining bodybuilder. Once you've made the mental commitment to give 100 percent effort in a particular day's workout, your body's energy reserves are what allow you to bomb and blitz your muscles with maximum training intensity for up to two hours at a time.

Merely living a regimented bodybuilding lifestyle and maintaining a healthy, muscle-building diet will quickly add to your energy reserves. But in this chapter, we are talking about developing the training energy reserves of a superman or superwoman without the use of drugs of any kind. All you'll use are a few new food supplements—many of which you've probably not heard of until now—that you will take on a daily basis to give yourself unbelievable energy levels.

NEARLY INSTANT ENERGY

One of the quickest and easiest ways to jack your energy up for a workout, or push it back up again in midworkout, is to pop three to five capsules of mixed free-form amino acids. Within 15–20 minutes you will experience a marked surge in training energy.

An even quicker surge of energy—one that you can feel within one or two minutes—can be had if you open the capsules and hold the powder within them under your tongue while the aminos are absorbed directly into your bloodstream. The effect is somewhat like the absorption of any sublingual prescription medicine. The taste of amino acid powder, however, is somewhat disagreeable, a bit like that of rotten eggs.

A problem with taking amino acids for an energy boost or for building muscle mass is their rather high cost. But once you experience the marked increase in energy a few seconds after putting the powder under your tongue or a few minutes after swallowing the capsules, you'll be convinced that the benefits definitely outweigh the cost of this supplement.

INOSINE

During the summer of 1983, coauthor Bill Reynolds went with Dr. Fred Hatfield, editor-in-chief of *Sports Fitness* magazine, to Moscow to study Soviet sports training techniques at the V. I. Lenin Central Institute for the Study of Sport and Physical Culture. Since Bill speaks Russian with relative ease, Fred and Bill set out to talk with some of the athletes to figure out the secrets that the local coaches weren't too happy about revealing in the seminars we attended.

Virtually every evening for two weeks, plying their subjects with copious quantities of vodka, Fred and Bill spent a lot of time swapping pins for the upcoming Los Angeles Olympics for 1980 Moscow Olympics pins. And they spent an inordinate amount of time learning which drugs were being used by guys like Vladimir Marchuk, who broke Vasili Alekseev's long-standing world record in the clean and jerk with a lift of nearly 580 pounds from the floor to straight arms' length overhead.

Marchuk had some incredible leg development (he did a triple Front Squat, rock bottom each rep, with 660 in one workout they watched), but he had a relatively weak-appearing upper body. At a height of about 5'10" and a body weight of 320 pounds, he was all stomach and legs. Oh, yeah, and he was only 20 years old when he eclipsed Alekseev's world record.

They wanted to know what drugs they were using, the quantities they were using, and how they were apparently beating the drug tests at international meets. They were also extremely interested in how these guys could recover between workouts and actually *improve* their strength and fitness levels when they were training up to three times per day with very heavy loads.

Recovery between workouts, it turned out, was part massage therapy, part heat treatments, and part the use of an injectable drug that when transliterated from the Cyrillic was called *iozin*. Fred quickly tracked down a non–Soviet bloc source of the drug, known in the Western world as inosine, to a manufacturer in Japan. They were making inosine tablets, but in 1983 the supplement wasn't available in North America.

Now inosine is sold in various combinations with other food elements in health food stores across the United States and Canada. The Great Earth chain of health food stores, for example, markets inosine in a compounded tablet called "Workout." By taking two to three tablets of this product (which works out to 400–600 milligrams of inosine) per day, you will notice an improvement in the speed with which you bounce back between workouts, as well as an improvement in aerobic capacity and general endurance. This isn't voodoo; it actually works!

When you go to a health food store next time, ask if it has any products with inosine as a component. You will probably be able to find it in most health food stores, and the cost isn't so prohibitive that you are unable to purchase a 30-day supply and give it a trial in your workouts. You should notice the difference in your training energy very quickly.

L-CARNATINE

An amino acid called L-carnatine also seems to have at least a mild effect on energy levels, and you can find this amino acid in health food stores, usually in combination with inosine. There is also a D-carnatine supplement often sold in combination with L-carnatine. However, D-carnatine can be toxic. Stick with the L-configuration of carnatine for an increase in energy.

DIMETHYLGLYCINE

Some supplement distributors carry bottles of DMG (dimethylglycine) with eyedroppers in them so that you can take three to five drops of DMG sublingually or in a glass of juice

20–30 minutes prior to a workout. Some bodybuilders feel that DMG improves aerobic endurance and general muscular endurance. We have conducted experiments with DMG at Gold's Gym in both Venice and Reseda, California, and most subjects have experienced no noticeable increase in energy from taking the suggested dosage of DMG 20–30 minutes before a training session. But when using five to ten times the recommended dosage, more than half of the subjects reported an increase in training endurance.

We suggest that you conduct your own experiments with various dosage levels of DMG and form your own conclusions about whether it is of sufficient value to continue its use.

B_{12} and B_{15}

Top bodybuilders have been using injectable vitamin B_{12} at least as far back as the late 1940s. I vividly recall talking with one of the true legends of the sport—a man who had won Mr. America, Mr. World, and Mr. Universe titles, and later won fame as an actor—when he told me that his favorite midworkout pick-me-up was an injection of testosterone mixed with B_{12}. And that was taking place back in 1950!

If you enjoy having needles jabbed into your rear end, you can inject B_{12}, but since it's water-soluble and quickly eliminated from your body, you will probably need a substantial injection virtually every day in order to feel a significant improvement in recovery ability between workouts. We personally prefer taking vitamin B_{12} in tablet form.

There's a considerable body of Soviet literature on Soviet experiments with pangamic acid (vitamin B_{15}) and I've read most of it. Regular injections or oral supplements of B_{15} appear to substantially improve capillarization and general blood circulation and thus augments aerobic capacity to a significant degree. Vitamin B_{15} tablets are widely available in health food stores.

When we mention injecting vitamins, please understand that we are *not* prescribing medicine. Vitamin B_{12} and vitamin B_{15} should only be prescribed by physicians and injected by medical personnel.

There are potential arguments for and against both oral and injectable dosages of vitamins B_{12} and B_{15}. Essentially, oral dosages are very safe but provide a somewhat limited amount of nutrient uptake. On the other hand, injectable dosages yield maximum nutrient uptake but present a minimal risk of infection from the injection equipment.

ADENISOTRIPHOSPHATE

Within your muscles, energy for maximum muscle contractions comes from the release of phosphate bonds when adenisotriphosphate (ATP) is reduced to adenisodiphosphate (ADP) is what exercise physiologists have named the Krebs Cycle.

ATP is naturally manufactured within your body, and there is experimental evidence that supplementally introduced ATP can increase the stores of this substance within muscle cells, thereby making significantly more energy available in the Krebs Cycle.

At the present time, ATP is available only for pharmaceutical use. In the future, it may be available as a food supplement. As such, it offers great potential for increased energy to fuel the vigorous muscle contractions of an all-out bodybuilding workout.

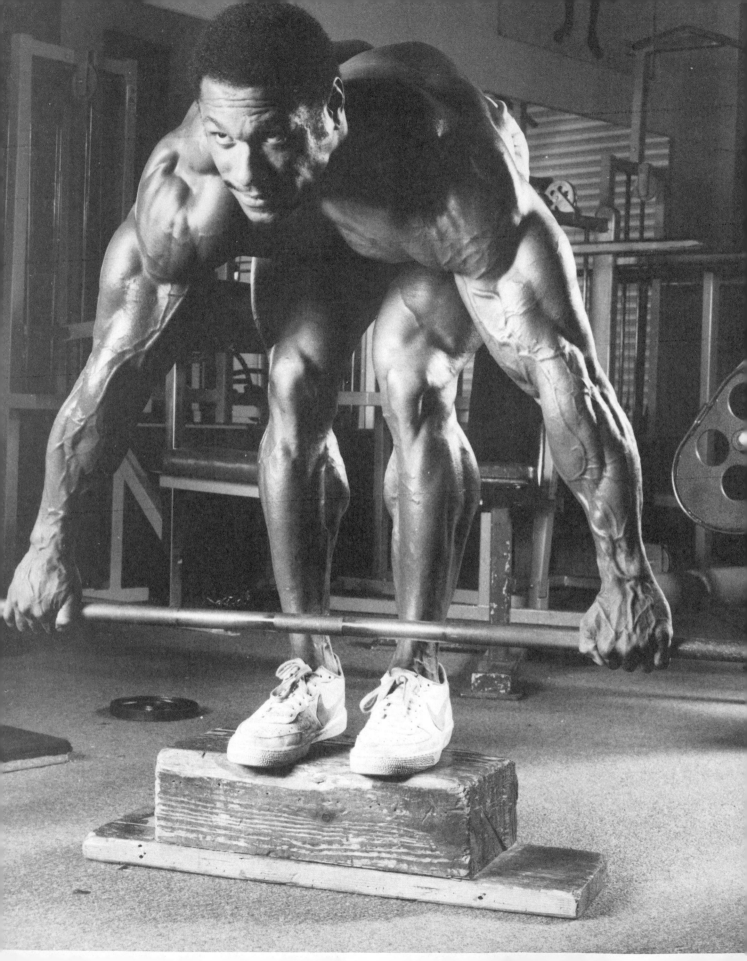

17
FOOD ALLERGIES

Have you ever suffered from mysterious water retention on-stage at a bodybuilding competition? Even though you've completely eliminated sodium from your diet for several days prior to your competition, you're holding enough water in your skin to look positively smooth onstage despite having a very low body fat percentage. If this is the case, it is very possible that you are suffering from a food allergy that is holding the excess water in your body.

Other common symptoms of food allergy are insomnia, muscle weakness, joint pains, muscle pains, arthritis, psychological depression, mental and physical lethargy, runny nose, asthma, chest congestion, sinus congestion, tachycardia, chronic fatigue, sore throat, stuffy ears, hyperactivity, irritability, restlessness, chronic fatigue, indifference, swelling of the extremities, hunger, binge eating, hives, rashes, pallor, dermatitis, acne, anxiety, aggressive behavior, panic attacks, and mood swings.

We aren't talking about severe allergies such as the nearly immediate hives some individuals suffer when they have eaten strawberries or some other food to which they are very allergic. Rather, we are talking about mild, insidious, almost unnoticeable allergies that have long-term negative effects on your body.

Just about everyone has eaten a food that was toxic to his or her body cells. These mildly allergenic foods are called cyto-toxic substances. *Cytotoxic* is a hybrid word coming from "cyto," meaning cell and "toxic," meaning poison. Therefore, cytotoxic foods are poisonous to the cells of your body. And everyone has at least several cytotoxic food allergies; some bodybuilders have at least 40–50 foods to which they are allergic. And it is these cytotoxic foods that retain water in the body and result in the long list of symptoms mentioned above.

There is a cytotoxic test in which blood is drawn, the white cells divided out of the blood with a centrifuge, and the white cells placed with tiny concentrates of every possible food. After two hours the white blood cells with each food are examined under a microscope. If the cells appear normal, you are not allergic to the food. If the cells are slightly distorted from their normal round appearance, you have a minor allergy to the food. And if the cells have been destroyed, you have a strong cytotoxic reaction to that particular food.

Although this is a relatively new test, many internal medicine specialists give it. Readers should consult their family physician for a referral to someone who gives the cytotoxic test in their area. It costs in the range of $300–$500. It's also relatively painless, and results are available after only one or two days.

It's highly probable that you will find that your favorite foods are the ones to which you are allergic. The reason for this is a subconscious process that occurs shortly after eating these foods. Cytotoxic foods act very much like cigarettes, and they can be just as addicting as tobacco.

No one who smokes ever actually enjoyed his or her first few cigarettes. But nicotine, which is a very powerful poison, enters the bloodstream after tobacco has been smoked, and the body must go into high gear to fight off this poison. The body going into high gear to fight off the nicotine gives a smoker the familiar lift, or rush, a person feels after smoking a cigarette. It takes about 15 minutes for the body to eliminate nicotine from the system, after which it returns to normal. And that's the point at which a smoker usually lights up again to get that little boost.

Cytotoxic foods work in a very similar manner. When you eat one, which is poison to your body's cells, your system must go into high gear to fight off the toxins. This gives you the same type of boost as a smoker gets from a cigarette. So, you very quickly become addicted to the cytotoxic foods in your diet, and that's the reason why you will probably find yourself addicted to the cytotoxic foods. All, or most, of your favorite foods will come up as cytotoxic when you take the test.

It takes only four to five days of avoiding cytotoxic foods to break the addiction and begin eliminating the negative symptoms caused by the poisonous foods. The elimination of retained water can be so dramatic that you might drop as many as eight to ten pounds of water weight in only one week, revealing muscularity that you didn't know you had. Done just before a competition, this loss of water due to the elimination of cytotoxic foods can make a tremendous difference in your appearance.

In terms of general health, however, it is best to maintain a diet free of cytotoxic foods year-round. Your training energy levels will be much higher, your mood more constant, and your general sense of well-being much higher. These are all factors which can make you a better bodybuilder, a winning bodybuilder. And winning is what our sport is all about when competing.

Even without taking a cytotoxic test, you can remove several of the most highly cytotoxic foods from your diet and improve your health and physical appearance dramatically. According to Dr. James Braly of Optimum Health Labs in Encino, California, "Most people are allergic to milk products and/or grains. Even if you can't take the test, it would be a good idea to drop these two food groups from your diet. If you do, you probably will notice a considerable improvement in your physical and mental health in only two or three weeks!"

We have tested Dr. Braly's advice at Gold's Gym and found it to be sound. However, it would be a good idea to also eliminate refined sugar from your diet since it is also a highly allergenic food. You can, however, consume rice when on a cytotoxic diet because rice is free from gluten, which is normally the component of grains and is allergenic.

You would be foolish to laugh off the information presented in this chapter. We have seen scores of men and women drastically improve their appearance, physical health, and mental health by following a cytotoxic diet. It does wonders for serious bodybuilders!

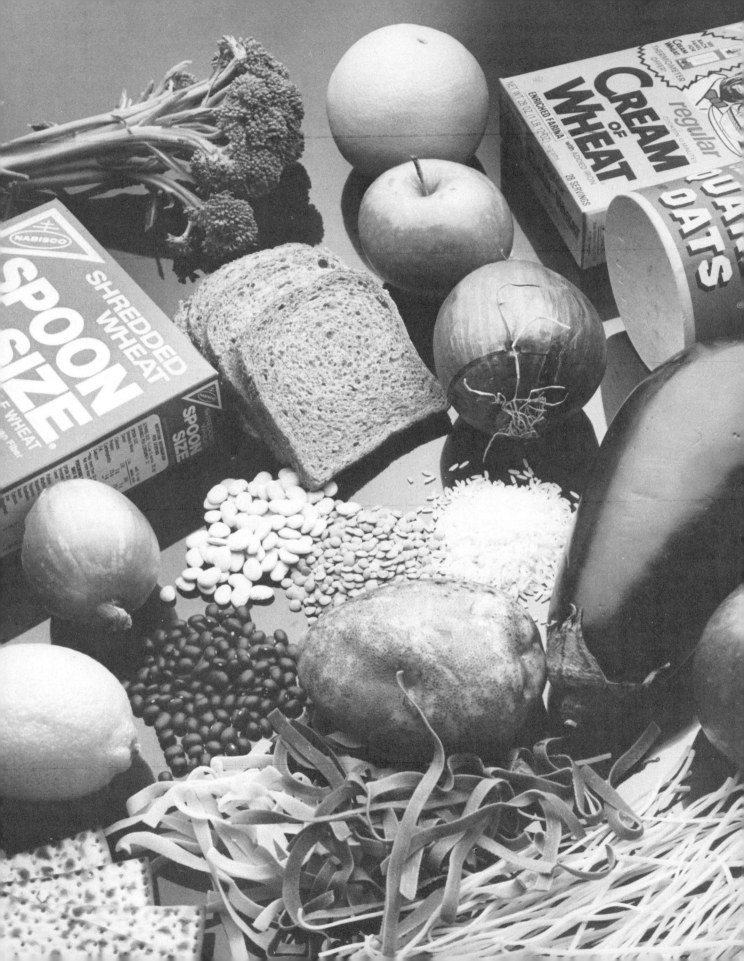

18
VEGETARIAN BODYBUILDING

Many bodybuilders have adopted a vegetarian lifestyle, avoiding flesh foods in their diet. The best-known vegetarian bodybuilders are Bill Pearl (Mr. America, Mr. USA, and four times Mr. Universe) and Andreas Cahling (IFBB Mr. International). But film Hercules Steve Reeves (Mr. America, Mr. World, and Mr. Universe) was also a vegetarian at least part of the time during his competitive bodybuilding career.

Very few bodybuilders are *vegans*, or individuals who consume only foods from vegetable sources—nuts, seeds, grains, fruit, and vegetables. Most bodybuilders are either *lacto-vegetarians* (who consume vegan foods and dairy products), or *lacto-ovo-vegetarians* (who consume the same foods as lacto-vegetarians, plus eggs). Both Bill Pearl and Andreas Cahling are lacto-ovo-vegetarians.

The health benefits of following a vegetarian lifestyle are well known. Vegetarians consume very low levels of saturated animal fats, so they have a low incidence of cardiac disease. A vegetarian diet is also conducive to optimum digestion, since animal flesh—particularly red meat—results in poor digestion. Because of the low fat content of vegetarian diets, it is usually much easier to control excess body fat stores when following a vegetarian diet. And there is considerable evidence that a vegetarian life-style contributes to longevity.

Many vegetarians avoid meat because it is a much more efficient process to consume vegetarian foods than the flesh of animals who themselves consume vegetable foods. An animal must consume approximately 10 times as much vegetarian food to produce protein food on a pound-for-pound basis. In other words, an acre of land can provide up to 10 times as much vegetable-source food as animal flesh.

Most uninformed bodybuilders would worry about the protein value of a vegetarian diet. But Bill Pearl notes, "A growing bodybuilder simply doesn't need 300–400 grams of protein per day to reach his potential. If the protein is from a natural source and is cooked as little as possible, the human body can survive very comfortably—even grow—on only 50–70 grams per day. Furthermore, this protein does not need to be meat, poultry, or fish but can come from vegetable or dairy foods. Beef is actually fairly low in protein because, once you remove all of the fiber, water, and uric acid from a prime steak, very little protein remains.

"If a bodybuilder is eating 300–400 grams of protein per day and is cutting his calories in preparation for a competition, he is bound to become fatigued and lethargic. As a result, the body must take protein and try to convert it to blood sugar to train on, a long process that consumes almost as much energy as it produces. If the bodybuilder doesn't have enough energy with which to train, why take in so much protein?

"The hypothetical bodybuilder I'm discussing would be far better off ingesting half or one-quarter of the protein he's eating, replacing the deleted meat calories with carbohydrate foods for energy. Carbohydrates are the body's preferred source of energy fuel, and anyone who eats an adequate supply of fresh fruit will have an abundance of training energy.

"There's absolutely no question that it is possible to build a high-class physique and be a vegetarian at the same time. Andreas Cahling did it, and I reached great condition at age 50 and later at age 55 doing the same thing. Another prime example is Roy Hilligen, a former Mr. America, who at 54 years of age, placed very high in the Mr. International competition. Roy has been a vegetarian as long as I've known him, and I met the guy about 1949 or 1950.

"Steve Reeves was about as close to being a vegetarian bodybuilder as anyone I have known, and he's one of the most revered athletes in bodybuilding history. Steve was almost exclusively a lacto-vegetarian, and he ate only minor amounts of meat. During the times I ate out with him, Reeves was always eating salads, avocados, fresh fruits, fresh vegetables, plus some occasional milk products."

If you fear that you won't make good bodybuilding gains following a vegetarian diet, you will be pleased to learn that Andreas Cahling actually made better gains after becoming a vegetarian: "Once I went completely lacto-vegetarian, I noticed I was feeling much better. My energy was higher and I was really blasting through my workouts. As a result, I began making unbelievable muscle gains all of the time while keeping my body fat levels lower than they'd ever been in the off-season. In five years, I added 25 pounds of solid muscle while following a vegetarian diet.

"I also used to be pretty irritable and touchy, particularly in the last few weeks before a competition when I was eating beef, chicken, and fish. Once I became a complete vegetarian—which was a gradual process—I became less and less jumpy. I even began to find it easier to fall asleep each night, which I couldn't do when I was eating flesh.

"To show you the dramatic effect of eating flesh—at least on my body—just eating a few pieces of sushi with a small amount of seafood in it can set me back to square one emotionally. Having lived in Japan for a year, I have a real taste for sushi, but in order to preserve my sanity and personal comfort I have to avoid eating this tasty delicacy!"

It is also possible to become very strong while following a vegetarian diet, but increased endurance is a more valuable benefit. Bill Pearl explains, "While they may not be as strong in terms of the amount of weight they can push, vegetarians have a great deal more endurance than the average bodybuilder. And just because a bodybuilder can push more weight doesn't mean he'll end up with more muscle. Weight counts, but so does the intensity of a workout, and intensity comes from how you feel the weight in an exercise and from how little you rest between sets when using maximum loads in all of your movements."

The Pearl of the Universe has been a vegetarian since about 1967. He recalls, "Back in the 1960s, I was working with the astronauts and company executives at North American Rockwell. I was telling these people all about good health. We were taking treadmill tests, and I was knocking these guys dead.

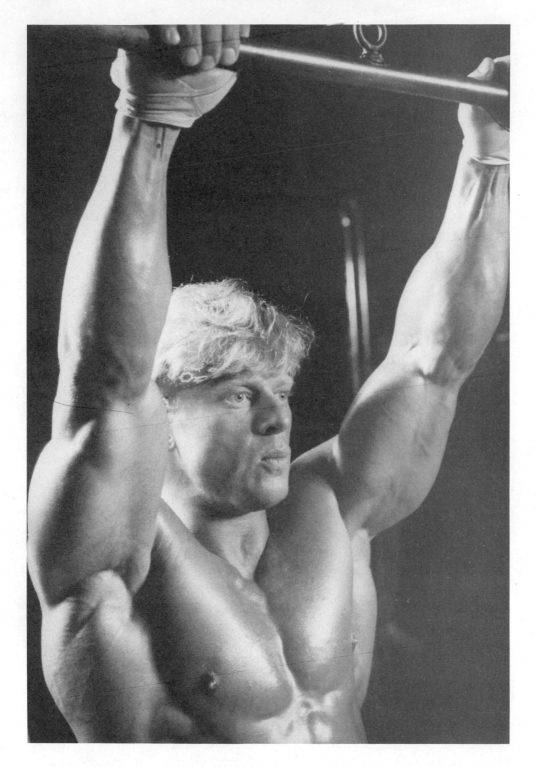

"One day—just as a lark—the doctor checked my cholesterol level. It was 307, an unbelievably high level, so my blood was running almost as thick as syrup through my veins. The doctor said, 'I don't give a damn how good you look, Bill, or how big your arm is. You're asking for trouble!' He went on to tell me I could die just as easily at 50 as anyone else, even though I felt I was in great shape. Naturally, that started me thinking.

"Because of bodybuilding, I was somewhat afraid to stop eating meats, but after the doctor told me this and I had successfully competed in the 1967 Pro Mr. Universe, I decided to change my eating habits. Becoming a lacto-vegetarian was my response to the situation, and except for a short period of meat eating before my last Universe in 1971, I've been a vegetarian since 1967. In 1971 I simply wasn't convinced I could do it again without meat, but at past 50 years of age and more than 15 years later I've reached great shape on a vegetarian diet.

"Vegetarian eating has had numerous positive effects on my body. My cholesterol gradually dropped down to a normal level of 198, and my blood pressure was markedly lowered. My pulse rate and other physiological processes are much better now, and overall I'm in better shape in my 50s than I was in my 20s.

"One of the most dramatic changes has been in my uric acid levels. My uric acid was so sky-high that every joint in my body ached; I could hardly move my hands. I actually thought I was getting arthritis!

"Today my energy levels are incredible, and I feel like a million dollars all of the time. There's nobody I've ever trained with whom I couldn't stay up with in a hard workout. My energy is greater than ever, and they don't need to knock off 15 cows a year just to keep me fed! Those cows are conceivably just as important on earth as any human being.

"The biggest change, however, has been in my attitude toward myself and my fellow man. Perhaps this sounds crazy, but I'm not nearly as aggressive as I have been in the past. There have been times in my life that I've wanted to go out and fight some guy for saying something that offended me. Or I'd scream and holler and really make an ass out of myself. Now I can catch myself smiling and trying to work out a problem. Vegetarianism has definitely had a mellowing effect on me."

Cahling's conversion to lacto-vegetarianism was relatively gradual: "I used to eat all of the flesh foods—beef, pork, chicken, turkey, lamb, and fish. My workouts were sluggish all of the time, but I didn't understand that the meat was causing my lethargy. My skin broke out, and I had extreme difficulty in getting ripped up for each of my competitions.

"Initially, I dropped beef and pork from my diet because they were so fatty that their high caloric content was keeping my own body fat levels too high. Oddly, I noticed that I also began to feel a little better, so I studied a few nutrition books. I was startled to learn how many steroids and other hormones were being shot into cattle and hogs to get their weight up. I didn't want that in my body, so I haven't touched beef or pork since then.

"About a year later I dropped poultry from my diet as well because chickens and turkeys are also pumped full of hormones. And as I dropped beef, pork, and poultry from my diet, I correspondingly increased my intake of fresh vegetables, fruit, milk products, grains, nuts, and seeds.

"Gradually, I ate fish less frequently each month and consumed progressively smaller quantities each time I ate fish. Finally, I was down to a sushi meal once every few weeks. I was feeling so good at this point and making such great gains from my sessions in the gym that I decided to go completely vegetarian. Believe me, it's the best decision of my life!"

Andreas disclosed his diet: "One of the staples of my diet is grilled cheese sandwiches. I take one slice of heavy, whole-grain bread and slap on a thick slab of raw goat cheese. Then I lightly toast this in the oven to melt the cheese into the bread. I might eat four or five of these open-faced sandwiches per day.

"Salads—especially those with a lot of sprouts, mushrooms, and tomatoes—are also a staple in my diet. I always eat these salads raw and without dressing. A medium-sized fresh salad is a gastronomical delight, and you won't even miss the dressing.

"I also eat a few nuts, some fruit, freshly squeezed fruit and vegetable juices, and perhaps some sunflower and pumpkin seeds during the day. Juices are very cleansing, especially green juices like celery, parsley, and spinach. I don't use steroids, but anyone who does would be a fool not to cleanse his body with juices periodically when on steroids.

"Because of my fresh and natural diet, I don't seem to need many food supplements. Just before a contest I'll take low-

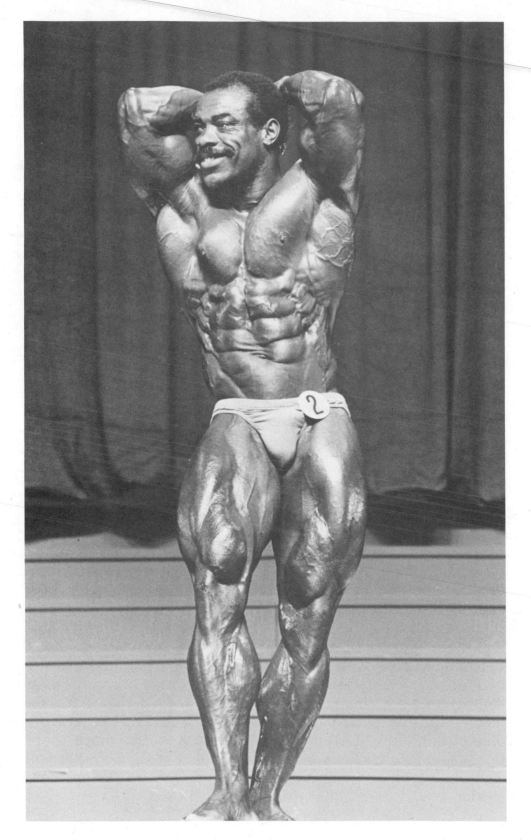

potency natural vitamins and minerals. You must be very careful in selecting supplements since so many today include petroleum derivatives. Read your labels carefully and, if you don't know a particular ingredient, don't buy the supplement."

Bill Pearl continues, "I don't presume to tell lacto-vegetarians what to eat. I can only tell you how I eat, and you can take it from there. When I get up at 3:45 in the morning—which suits my life-style—I might have a cup of mint tea as a perker-upper. Once back at home from the gym, I might have a cheese omelette or five or six eggs prepared in some other way. I might also have a little cottage cheese, some heavy type of bran bread with butter, and another cup of tea.

"For lunch I'll have a large fresh salad, putting the widest possible variety of salad ingredients into it. The only dressing might be a small amount of oil and vinegar.

"At night my wife will cook up some type of a soufflé, or perhaps a casserole. I'll have another fresh salad and for dessert maybe some yogurt or fruit. My supplements include a good B complex, C, E, kelp, and zinc. I think that after the age of 40–45 zinc is very important for gland health. And that's my total diet."

For an ill-informed bodybuilder, a vegetarian diet can raise difficulties when traveling or eating out. Cahling explains how he overcomes this problem: "I travel quite a bit to compete, give training seminars, present posing exhibitions, and to take care of my swim wear business dealings. I can always find a good salad bar at my hotel and even order a vegetarian meal on the plane if I call ahead. Still, I carry food with me on trips for snacks and to tide me over in emergencies when I can't find the right restaurant at which to eat. For a day, cheese will keep without spoiling, so I pack a little of my favorite goat's milk cheese. Favorite nonperishable foods that I carry are various seeds and nuts, plus a few slices of flourless bread. This technique works really well for me."

You need not become a total vegetarian to reap many of the benefits of a vegetarian lifestyle. Simply avoiding flesh foods at some meals—perhaps even entirely avoiding meat certain days—will give you many of the benefits of a full vegetarian diet, but in reduced magnitude. If you wish to read more about the actual mechanics of a vegetarian diet, we suggest that you read Paavo Airola's book, *Are You Confused?* (Contemporary, 1971).

Bill Pearl sums up the vegetarian bodybuilder's attitude toward his dietary life-style: "Once you are eating as a vegetarian, you can't be swayed away from it by anyone or anything, regardless of the situation. If a person offered me $50,000 to eat a steak, I'd tell him to stick it in his pocket. What's the sense of making a commitment if you're not committed? I'm a firm believer in sticking to my convictions, and I'm committed to following a vegetarian lifestyle for the remainder of my years!"

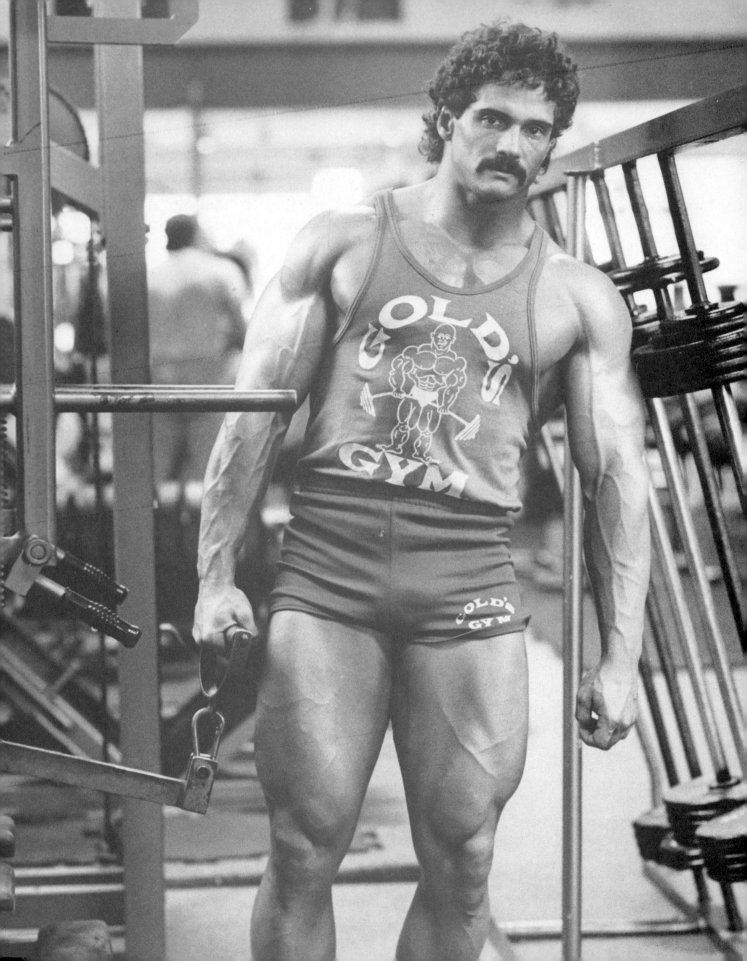

19
DETOXIFYING YOUR BODY

Given the widespread use of anabolic drugs and the insidious effect of environmental pollution on the body, you will probably be happy to know that there are nutritional methods of detoxifying your body. Through intelligent use of various food supplements and by fasting, you can significantly reduce the harmful effects of drug use and pollution on your liver, kidneys, and other internal organs.

WATER

One of the best detoxifying agents is pure water, notably distilled water. Without adequate intake of pure water each day, your kidneys can become clogged with environmental pollutants and other toxins. By adequate water intake, we mean pure water unencumbered by coffee grounds, tea leaves, artificial sweeteners, and so forth.

Chapter 6 was devoted to a discussion of the values of water in your diet. You should consume at least eight to ten glasses of distilled water, or water from natural springs, each day. Many large male bodybuilders consume a gallon or more of pure water each day, which helps them to keep their kidneys from being clogged with toxins.

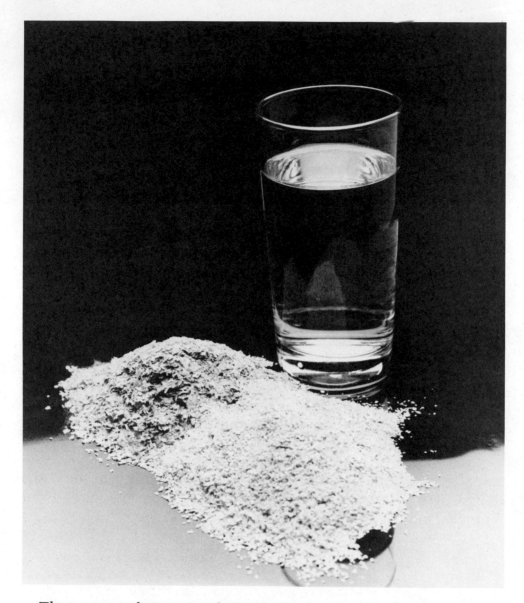

There are also several vitamin supplements that have a detoxifying action on your body. Chief among these is vitamin C, which is well known as an antioxidant. Expert nutritionists advise an ascorbic acid intake of 1,000–3,000 milligrams per day for men and women who live in large industrial cities where pollution can have a deleterious effect on human health.

Vitamin A, which is oil soluble and thus storable in your body, is another detoxification agent. A daily intake of at least 15,000 units of vitamin A is recommended to counteract toxin build-ups. And when you are suffering from an infection, such as a cold or flu, you can double or triple your intake of vitamin A to help ward off the infection.

Vitamin E in doses of at least 400 i.u. per day can also have an antioxidant action in your body. However, the most important detoxification agents are vitamins A and C. Other helpful vitamins include B_1, B_2, and niacin. And selenium and zinc are the most helpful minerals in keeping your body free of toxins.

The foregoing vitamins and minerals can be taken individually or in combinations found in health food stores. One excellent combination of the major detoxification agents can be found in a supplement called Nutrox, which is distributed by Integrated Health, Inc. in Santa Monica, California. We use this supplement ourselves and highly recommend it to all bodybuilders.

FASTING

Health-conscious individuals have known of the cleansing benefits of fasting since ancient times. But in today's modern society, fasting is sometimes looked upon as a faddist activity. Still, fasting is probably the single best tool for detoxifying your body.

Vegetarian bodybuilder Andreas Cahling comments on the values and procedures of fasting: "Man is a slow learner. Neither nature itself nor irrefutable history seems able to convince him that sometimes *not* eating is healthful. Instead, bodybuilders continue to gorge themselves with every food item available and suffer from all sorts of problems as a result—protein overdoses, hypoglycemia, obesity—not to mention that they bring their muscularity quest to a grinding halt.

"Yet all of the evidence is there. Wild animals are not only able to heal themselves without drugs, but they do not suffer from being overweight. Since creation, nature has been beating us over the head with the fact that animals have always instinctively avoided food when ill. To these 'lower' animals, a decreased appetite during disease is an alarm signal, telling them to 'starve a fever.' Still, we can't seem to grasp that. We continue to flaunt our favorite maxim of conceit: 'Man is the only rational animal.' Of course, that's man's definition, not animal's.

"As if nature weren't qualified enough as a teacher, we've also failed to grasp the message of thousands of years of history. Even before the age of tribal medicine men, fasting was used to cure diseases and rejuvenate the body. Hippocrates, the father of medicine, recommended fasting, while Socrates and Plato used fasting to obtain physical and mental highs. The Greeks were not alone in their respect of fasting; philosophers and yogis of the Orient—known for longevity and mental acuity, as well as spiritual consciousness—practice fasting.

"The logic behind fasting is convincing. Let's start with Hans Selye, the renowned Canadian physician and author. Selye's concept is basic: 'A person is as young or old as his smallest vital component, the cell; therefore, to maintain youth and health, our bodies must constantly be producing more cells to replace dead cells. Unfortunately, when we allow toxins and other waste products to build up in our bodies, these products interfere with the growth of new cells. To resist aging, we must not only promote the building of healthy new cells, but we must also eliminate aged and dead cells from our bodies as quickly as possible.

"Fasting becomes necessary when there is no longer an effective means of rapidly clearing out cellular waste to provide a healthful environment for new cells.

"How can something as simple as abstinence from food provide such positive results? During a prolonged fast—more than three days—the body lives on its own tissue. Sounds dangerous, doesn't it? Yet, ironically, fasting is probably the most healthful road you can take toward bodybuilding success. Let me tell you why.

"The secret of fasting's effectiveness is that the body is selective in the use of its own cells. First, to satisfy its nourishment needs, it starts breaking down and burning the cells which are diseased, degenerated, old, or dead. During a fast, the body feeds on the most unclean and inferior material in the body, such as fat deposits, tumors, and so forth. Cells from important body organs, the nervous system and the brain, will not be used. The advantage of this process to a bodybuilder is obvious: with the wide use of steroids today and a prepossessing lust for getting ripped, the fast is a means of achieving new muscle tissue, flushing out toxins, and rejuvenating strength and cells.

"It's difficult to believe that your body can actually build new cells faster when you limit your nutrients, but it's a physiological fact. Fasting requires a faith in your body's ability to take care of itself. In fact, if you give it a chance, your body will do a better job of maintaining its own health than you can.

"Even though no protein is consumed during a fast, your blood protein level will remain normal. That's because the protein in your body will be converted from one form to another in order to satisfy specific needs. Amino acids—the building blocks of protein—can be reused time after time to build new cells.

"Waste products and other toxins reduce your body's efficiency, so your objective should be to get rid of them as quickly as possible. When you fast, organs such as lungs, kidneys, and liver are relieved of their waste loads, freeing them for higher work capacities. That's why you experience renewed energy during a fast. And remember, there's no reason to cut back on your workouts; in fact, you can approach them with renewed vigor.

"Mental attitude can mean the difference between success and failure during a fast. Just remember that there is no relationship between forced starvation and voluntary abstinence from food. Forced starvation carries with it uncertainty and fear, which has a paralyzing effect on body functions and can damage your health.

"However, if you approach fasting with a confidence and a full understanding of its benefits, your body, in turn, will respond to this positive attitude.

"Even symptoms that seem adverse are actually beneficial results of a fast. For example, after the first two or three days, you might experience a slight headache and light dizziness. Your skin might even break out. But this just means that the amount of toxins expelled during a fast can be 10 times the normal level. Try to ignore your anxiety and be proud of the fast's cleansing effect.

"For optimum bodybuilding benefits, you should go on a short fast about three months before your next contest. This will stimulate your body's natural anabolism for increased muscle tissue production, while bringing out your cuts and giving you new training energy and motivation.

"If you have been using steroids or other drugs, their effects may linger after you stop taking them, so allow about two months for your body to return to normal before initiating a fast to cleanse it.

"Since food supplements can only be assimilated in combina-

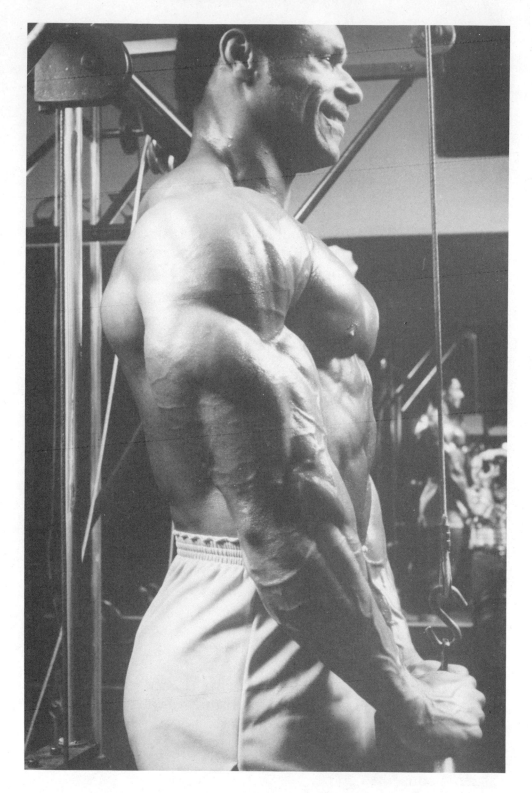

tion with food, they should also be curtailed. During a fast, you would simply be wasting them.

"If you've never fasted before, or if you plan on fasting only with water, definitely see your physician first. A fruit and vegetable juice fast for a limited time, on the other hand, presents no danger and is something that you can begin tomorrow.

"Some might claim that a fast on juices rather than water is not a 'real' fast, but it's actually the superior one. Juices accelerate the body's cleansing capacity by supplying necessary minerals and ionic charges.

"To prepare your body for a fast, begin with a two- or three-day diet consisting of only raw fruit and vegetables as well as juices. Eat fruit one meal and vegetables the next; do not mix fruit and vegetables at the same meal, because each requires different enzymes for proper digestion.

"On the fourth day, begin your juice diet and remain on it for four to six days. Gradually, feelings of hunger will disappear. Drink as much juice as you can because this both increases the cleansing action and subdues hunger. Carrot, celery, apple, and watermelon juices are all excellent.

"The famous 'health doctor' Otto F. Buchinger said, 'Even an idiot can fast, but only a wise man knows how to break a fast.' In other words, the great benefits of a fast can be sabotaged if your return to a solid food diet is not carried out properly.

"I offer three simple rules for returning to a more normal diet. First, eat small amounts of food when you begin to consume solids. Second, eat slowly and chew the food thoroughly. And third, gradually return to a normal diet.

"During this transition period of two or three days, your diet should consist of only raw fruit and vegetables. Then gradually include other foods.

"Perhaps the most important rule of all is to completely avoid all coffee and drugs. A fast highly sensitizes your body to drugs, and the smallest amount can seriously damage you.

"Try fasting. Your first experience will be an astounding one. The fast will not only change the composition of your body but also your mind. Rather than maintaining a body composed of diseased cells and painful poisons, you'll have a body consisting of pure, natural organic nutrients and fresh, new muscle tissue. And rather than having a mind of pure, self-limiting ego, you'll have a fresh, clear brain power. And that's the only way to the top!"

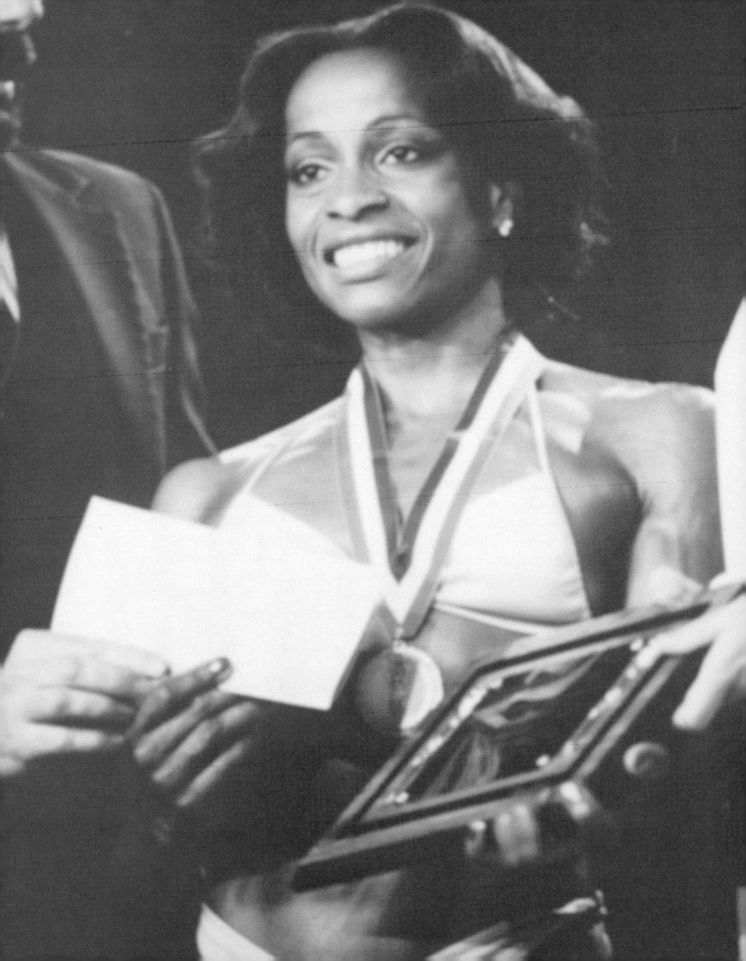

20
THE MENTAL SIDE OF BODYBUILDING NUTRITION

As the twig is bent, so grows the tree. As the mind is oriented in bodybuilding, so goes the body.

"In both training and nutrition, the body follows the course your mind has set," states Tom Platz (Mr. Universe). Every champion bodybuilder training at Gold's Gym would agree with Tom's assertion.

In a very real sense, you can *will* your body to look a certain way, then cause it to reach that appearance through specific dietary and training practices. It takes a deep mental commitment to establish the nutritional willpower required to totally rework your body the way a once-overweight Dawn Marie Gnaegi did enroute to building a world-class physique, or the way a once painfully thin Lou Ferrigno did in muscling up to become the biggest Mr. Universe in the history of the sport and a well-known television star.

At 5'1" in height, Dawn Marie Gnaegi once weighed a pudgy 170 pounds, a majority of the excess baggage situated between her waist and knees. With fierce determination in the gym, she progressively intensified her bodybuilding workouts. Steadfastly, she burned more and more calories pedaling a stationary bike, running, and taking aerobics classes. And with a will of iron, she gradually reduced the total number of calories she consumed each day.

Within a couple of years, a national-caliber physique had emerged, like a beautiful statue emerges from what was once a raw block of marble. Coming from nowhere, Dawn Marie was runner-up in the middleweight class at both the American and National Championships during 1983. She was competing at a sensationally muscular 114 pounds, nearly 60 pounds less than she had once weighed.

During 1984, Dawn Marie Gnaegi became the U.S. Middleweight Champion and again placed second in the American Championships after a draining struggle to make the 114-pound middleweight class limit one final time. She now competes successfully in the pro ranks with her voluptuously muscled and still super-ripped 123-pound physique.

"It takes willpower to lose fat weight," reveals Gnaegi. "Dictionaries define willpower as energetic determination. And it took a great deal of willpower to turn my lifestyle into that of a world-class bodybuilder, and hence my shapeless body into that of a champion bodybuilder.

"How did it all start for me? It started with visions, and I'm not talking about the Jean Dixon type of vision. I recall standing in front of a full-length mirror remembering always having been plump. But on this particular day I realized I was no longer plump; I was fat. I stared into the mirror for some time, realizing that I'd always be fat if I didn't do something about the problem immediately.

"The energetic determination I would use to change my body and lifestyle burst into flame at that moment, fueled by visions of how I used to look and how I soon wished to appear. That day's vison of becoming a lean, athletic, healthy woman came true for me, because I wanted it to happen and *made* it happen.

"I now notice the physical appearance of people more than I used to, and I see a lot of overweight men and women. Not everyone is cut out to be a champion bodybuilder, but everyone *should* be concerned with good health. Being overweight is definitely *not* healthy.

"Breaking bad habits isn't easy, and it requires a great deal of willpower to do it. Don't we all love to eat? I certainly do! Be honest with yourself, however. Don't we all love to look good? Of course! And that's where desire and willpower come into play."

Lou Ferrigno had the opposite problem that Dawn Marie Gnaegi had. He needed to mentally drive himself to train with progressively heavier poundages and condition his mind to accept the logic of eating five to six protein-rich meals per day rather than the normal two to three that he ate before taking up bodybuilding. This is what it took for Lou to fill out his bean-pole frame sufficiently to merely appear normally athletic, let alone to win two IFBB Mr. Universe titles and become internationally famous for the massive physique he displayed as the "Incredible Hulk" on television.

While there are significant numbers of overweight young men and women taking up bodybuilding, the vast majority of new bodybuilders are in the sport to gain muscular body weight. And there is no better method to reach this goal than heavy bodybuilding training and proper nutrition. That's why so many athletes from other sports—particularly football—have taken to pumping iron to gain functional weight and greater power.

"I can really identify with underweight teenagers who have decided to get into the gym and work at improving their appearance," says Lou Ferrigno. "I was one of them. When I began training in my mid-teens, I was already nearly six feet tall and weighed only 135 pounds. To say I was skinny would have been an understatement.

"It wasn't difficult for me to mentally accept the workouts, but it took considerable psychological conditioning to gradually increase my food consumption. Like most underweight youngsters, I was seldom hungry, and it was actually a chore to force down the nutritional meals I needed in order to gain weight. You can train fantastically hard and still fail to make gains if you don't eat enough high-quality protein and sufficient calories to accommodate your body's needs.

"If you are underweight, make up your mind that nothing is going to stop you. And don't let anyone or anything stop your progress to your goal. That's the way I did it. Build up an overwhelming desire to become big and muscular, set clearly defined goals, and be consistent in both training and diet. With a complete psychological, physical, and nutritional approach like this, you'll definitely succeed in packing on the beef you're after."

MIND-SET

You're the only person who can make up your mind to succeed as a bodybuilder. Only you can discipline yourself to follow a low-calorie diet if you need to lose body fat. Only you can be certain that you consume sufficient protein-rich meals to increase muscular body weight if you are underweight. Only you can push yourself away from the table when you are overweight. Only *you* are responsible for whether you improve.

When you make up your mind to follow a certain dietary course, set it fairly. Don't be the wishy-washy type who's dieting for a contest six days a week and pigging out on ice cream the seventh. This type of bodybuilder never succeeds. He or she is doomed to always coming out second-best, or even to never making any progress at all. Is this what you want?

What we're talking about here is *commitment*, and when you make a *commitment*, your mind becomes set on reaching the goal you have set. And without this mind-set it becomes difficult, if not impossible, to achieve the goal you have set for yourself.

Bill Pearl (Mr. America, Mr. USA, and four times Mr. Universe) noted, "Once I had set the date of an upcoming competition or exhibition firmly in my mind, it was almost as if my body began to improve at the exact rate of speed it would take to reach perfect condition on the exact date I needed to be in peak shape. I'm sure that making up my mind to be in top condition on a set date programmed my subconscious mind to help me to more easily reach that type of shape."

GOAL SETTING

Goal setting is one of the best ways to mentally focus your energies on accomplishing any bodybuilding task. Goal setting in bodybuilding nutrition gives your mind and body an exact road map to success so that you don't waste time taking detours or going up blind alleys.

It's essential that you set both large, long-term goals and small, short-term goals. And these short-term goals should, when accomplished, gradually walk you step by step up to each long-range goal.

You will find it mind-boggling to confront yourself with a

long-term goal such as gaining 20 pounds of solid muscle, or losing 30 pounds of body fat. But if you divide this large goal up into one-pound goals, you will be able to forget the big pie-in-the-sky goal and focus on the more manageable one-pound goal. Each pound of muscle gained or pound of fat lost is one more step toward your primary goal, and once you add up enough steps, you will have reached a long-range goal.

When you set goals for yourself, be sure that they are both realistic and high enough to push you to excel. There's no point in a man expecting to gain 30 pounds of muscle in a year, because eight to ten pounds of lean body mass is the most anyone can expect to gain in one year. There's also no point in a woman expecting to gain eight to ten pounds in a year when four to five is the most she can expect to gain. But a man *should* set his goal to gain the full ten pounds, a woman the full five pounds.

Although you should do everything in your power to reach each goal, it is no sin to fall short of your target goal from time to time. Goals are meant to extend you in your efforts to reach each one, but it's not at all uncommon for a bodybuilder to overestimate the abilities of his or her own body to improve.

Once you reach a long-term goal (usually set at one-year intervals), set a new one. Think of these long-term goals as islands stretching across a lake, with short-term goals being stepping stones between each island. By properly setting goals, you will discover that day by day and step by step, you are getting better.

VISUALIZATION

Visualization is one of the best mental tools you have at your disposal to guarantee that your training and dietary efforts and practices are improving your physique at an optimum rate of speed. It is really nothing more than a directed form of daydreaming, but it's the way in which you can program your subconscious mind to make those decisions that make it easier to reach the visualized goals. The process is a lot like a young man or woman dreaming for years about becoming a physician, fantasizing about the occupation to the point where they almost begin to live the occupation. When there's this much involvement in a fantasy, the subconscious mind makes it much easier to stay up late at night for years studying medicine.

In some ways, an accomplished bodybuilder must be as dedicated as a medical student. It takes as much persistence, as many years of preparation, and often as many hours per day of involvement as the study of medicine in order to become a successful bodybuilder. So, it's little wonder that you, a serious bodybuilder, would need visualization to reach your goals.

Psychologists call visualization *self-actualization*. It is literally the process of making your dreams come true through hard work, aided by the preprogrammed subconscious mind. So, how do you program your subconscious mind?

Visualization is best practiced at night when you are in bed preparing to fall asleep. The technique is used best when it's dark, you are completely relaxed, and there is no chance of interruption, three conditions that are met when you are lying in bed with the lamp out preparing to sleep. It must be practiced virtually every day in order for it to be maximally effective, but you will find the process so pleasurable that you'll look forward to doing it each day.

When you are fully relaxed, begin to build a visual image of how you wish to soon appear. This image should be almost like a movie film projected against a screen formed by the backs of your eyelids.

Make the image as clear and as realistic as possible. Visualize every ridge and valley of muscle across your back, shoulders, chest, arms, abdominals, and legs. Visualize the tracery of large arteries and smaller branching veins flowing with life-giving blood. Visualize how thin your skin is, so that it vividly reveals the deep, contest-ready muscularity beneath it.

Normally, this is as far as most bodybuilders take the visualization process, and it will be effective when used regularly in this manner. But psychologists have concluded that you can receive many times more benefit from the visualization procedure if you can involve more than just the visualized sense of sight. Can you think of ways to include the sensations of touch, hearing, smell, and taste?

Allow us to give you a few hints about how to do this. The sense of touch can come into play quite easily as you imagine the feel of your huge, ripped-up muscles extending and then powerfully contracting under heavy loads during a workout.

And the sense of hearing is as easy as imagining the sound of plates rattling on an Olympic bar as you do heavy movements in your bodybuilding training program.

Taste and smell come easily into play in a dietary scenario. We're sure you can easily imagine the flavor and aroma of a skinned chicken breast that has just been broiled over a charcoal fire.

If you properly use visualization and the other mental techniques discussed in this chapter, we're sure that you will find it much easier to consume the right foods during various stages of your diet. And this ability to eat correctly in a bodybuilding sense is 50 percent of the battle when you are attempting to become a champion in our sport.

THE OPTIMUM BODYBUILDER'S DIET

Based on all of the research we have done to complete this book, we have arrived at the following 10 elements of an optimum bodybuilder's diet:

1. All foods should be prepared in as fresh a state as possible in order to retain a maximum number of nutrients, particularly digestive enzymes that are quickly lost as a piece of fruit or meat is left too long in the refrigerator.

2. Along the same line as the rule 1, avoid processed foods—any foods that have been packaged, canned, bottled, or frozen.

3. Consume smaller and more frequent meals each day, four to six rather than the normal two to three. Be sure each meal contains approximately 20 grams of pure protein, the most any bodybuilder can hope to digest and assimilate each meal. Milk and eggs have protein of the highest biological quality, while poultry and fish have protein that is both of high biological quality and easy to digest and assimilate into muscle tissue.

4. Choose protein supplements according to which ones are most assimilable into muscle tissue in your body. Protein supplements with milk, egg whites, and animal organs have the highest PERs and are optimally assimilable. And although they are rather expensive, free-form amino acids are the most assimilable form of protein supplement. On the other end of the scale, protein supplements derived from vegetable sources

(soybeans, sesame seeds, etc.) are of much lower biological quality.

5. Eat one-half to three-quarters of a gram of high-quality protein per pound of body weight each day. Although some misguided bodybuilders consume two grams of protein per pound of body weight, they don't receive any more benefit than those athletes who eat only one-half gram of protein. They simply clog up their digestive systems and grow fat from the excess calories they ingest.

6. Use one to two multipacks of vitamins, minerals, and trace elements per day *with meals* as insurance against progress-halting nutritional deficiencies. Individual supplemental vitamins and minerals are optional and should be chosen over a period of time through trial and error.

7. Base carbohydrate consumption primarily on complex carbohydrate foods (e.g., potatoes, rice, other grains, and vegetables) that yield a sustained, long-lasting flow of training energy. Simple carbohydrate foods (e.g., sugar-laden junk foods and fruit) result in a short-term burst of energy. Fruit is best used just before a workout, and/or in midworkout when energy reserves have been depleted.

8. Restrict the amount of fat in your diet, and keep consumption of animal fats as low as possible due to their high caloric and cholesterol counts. Specifically avoid pork, beef, full-fat milk products, and egg yolks.

9. Drink plenty of distilled or purified water, or mountain spring water, each day. Men should drink a minimum of eight to ten glasses of water per day (women should drink six to eight) to help flush toxins from your body and keep your system purified.

10. Eat for nutrition, not for taste. Although most top bodybuilders have occasional cravings for ice cream and other junk foods, they eat primarily for the nutritional content of each meal, making the taste of various foods irrelevant.

BON APPETIT

Throughout this Gold's Gym nutrition book we have emphasized that nutrition is at least half of the battle to become a champion bodybuilder. And we have given you all of the nutritional information you need in order to ultimately build a physique with exceptional muscle mass and outstanding muscle density and muscularity. But it's totally up to you to use this information to improve your physique; we simply can't eat your meals for you. We *know* you can do it, so go for the gold the Gold's Gym way!

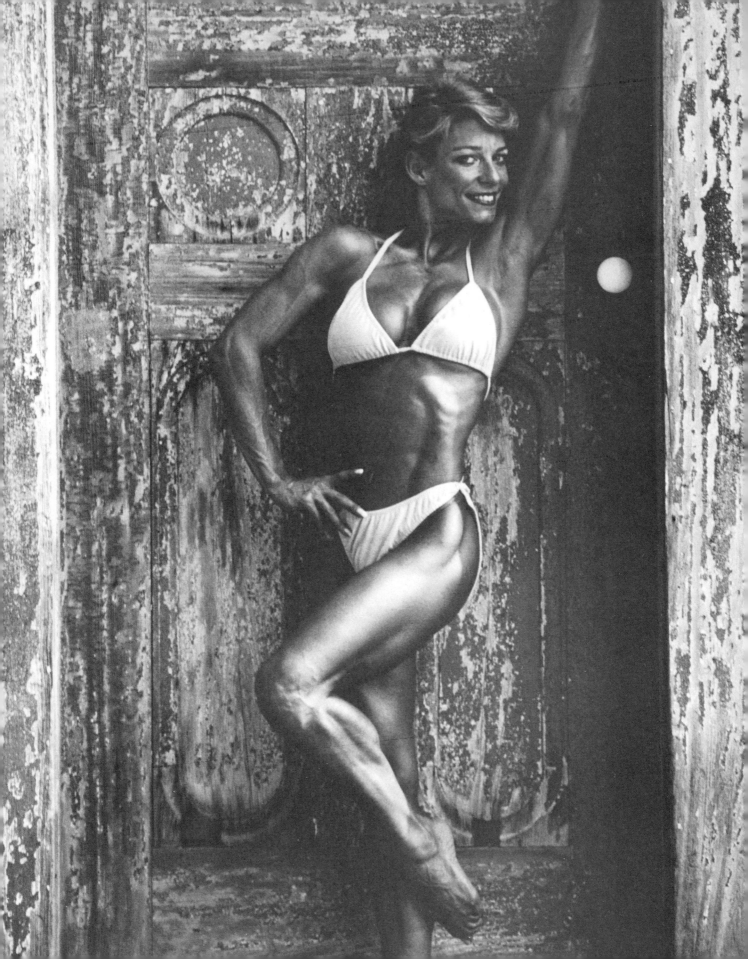

APPENDIX
THE CHAMPIONS'
FAVORITE RECIPES

ORANGE WHIP

DEBBIE BASILE (AMERICAN LIGHTWEIGHT CHAMPION)

Ingredients:
1½ envelopes unflavored gelatin
3½ cups orange juice
3 tablespoons lemon juice
2 tablespoons frozen apple juice
2 packets artificial sweetener

In a small mixing bowl, soften gelatin in ½ cup of orange juice. Heat the remaining orange juice, bringing it to a boil. Add this to the gelatin mixture and stir until gelatin is dissolved. Add apple juice, lemon juice, and artificial sweetener. Chill until the mixture begins to thicken. Beat with an electric mixer until fluffy. Chill, then serve.

Makes six servings. Each serving contains the following:
Calories: 400   Carbs(g): 62   Protein(g): 3   Fat(g): —

BECKLES' SPECIAL BREAD

ALBERT BECKLES (WORLD PRO GRAND PRIX CHAMPION, SECOND-
PLACE FINISHER, MR. OLYMPIA)

Ingredients:
4 eggs
4 cups water
1 teaspoon nutmeg
1 teaspoon cinnamon
½ cup honey
½ pound coconut
1 pound raisins
2 cups powdered lecithin
2 level teaspoons baking powder
2½ pounds whole-wheat flour

In a large mixing bowl, use a wooden spoon to combine
eggs, one cup of water, spices, and honey. Mix together until
blended well. Add another two cups of water, coconut,
raisins, lecithin, and baking powder. Stir so that all
ingredients are mixed together. Lastly, add one more cup of
water and sift in flour while mixing together one last time.
Place dough in equal amounts in four greased, nonstick loaf
baking pans. Bake at 300 degrees for one hour, or until top is
golden brown. (Be sure to check frequently.) Remove from
oven and allow to cool. Bread that is not needed can be
frozen.

Makes six loaves. Each loaf contains the following:
Calories: 1,565   Carbs(g): 130   Protein(g): 45   Fat(g):

RATATOUILLE

LAURA COMBES (OVERALL AMERICAN CHAMPION)

Ingredients:
1 onion
2 cloves garlic
¼ cup olive oil
1 egg plant (peeled)
1 large zucchini (or two small ones)
2 green peppers
6 tomatoes (or one big can of drained tomatoes)
salt (Laura uses Morton's Lite Salt, which is lower in sodium)
pepper
sweet basil

Sauté chopped onions and garlic in olive oil. Add all of the vegetables, which have been cut into small pieces. Add salt (very little), pepper, and basil to taste and simmer in a covered pot until all of the vegetables are soft (about 35 minutes). Remove cover and simmer until contents of pot have thickened. This dish can be served hot or cold (with lemon to taste). I personally prefer it cold on hot days.

Makes two large servings. Each serving contains the following:
Calories: 440   Carbs(g): 40   Protein(g): 7   Fat(g): 28

PRECONTEST-STYLE SWEET 'N' SOUR CHICKEN
ELAINE CRAIG (APPLE CUP CHAMPION)

Ingredients:
½ pound chicken breast (skinned and cut into bite-sized
    chunks)
1 green bell pepper (sliced)
½ onion (sliced)
1 carrot (sliced diagonally)
1 piece celery (sliced diagonally)
⅛ cup soy sauce
⅛ cup water
2 packets artificial sweetener

Cook chicken in nonstick skillet. Chicken is cooked when it
turns white in color. Add remaining ingredients and cook for
five minutes, stirring frequently.

Makes one serving. Each serving contains the following:
Calories: 345   Carbs(g): 27   Protein(g): 41   Fat(g): 9

TERIYAKI CHICKEN
DIANA DENNIS (OVERALL NATIONAL CHAMPION, CALIFORNIA PRO GRAND PRIX CHAMPION)

Ingredients:
1 4-ounce chicken breast (boned and skinned)
¼ cup bottled teriyaki sauce (the brand found in health food stores is sweetened with honey rather than sucrose)

Marinate chicken for three hours in teriyaki sauce. Broil for four minutes each side and serve with steamed rice. I use this dish throughout my contest preparation cycle because the sauce contains no sugar.

Makes one serving. Each serving contains the following:
Calories: 270   Carbs(g): 38   Protein(g): 18   Fat(g): 4

SCRAMBLED OMELETTE

CORINNA EVERSON (OVERALL NATIONAL CHAMPION, TWICE MS. OLYMPIA)

Ingredients:
6 egg whites (large)
1 thinly sliced onion
1 finely chopped zucchini
½ teaspoon garlic powder
2 tablespoons water

In a large nonstick skillet, heat onion and zucchini over low heat. Add water. Cook until onion is clear, stirring often. Add egg whites and garlic powder. Cook until eggs are done. Sprinkle with parmesan cheese and serve with one slice whole-wheat toast.

Makes one serving. Each serving contains the following:
Calories: 198   Carbs(g) : 20   Protein(g): 24   Fat(g): —

APPLE DESSERT

JEFF EVERSON (MIDWEST CHAMPION, AMERICAN MIXED PAIRS CHAMPION)

Ingredients:
1 medium-sized green apple (cut into small pieces)
¼ cup chopped walnuts
1 teaspoon margarine
1½ ounces raisins
1 packet artificial sweetener
ground cinnamon

Using a nonstick skillet, melt margarine over medium heat. Add apples and chopped walnuts, stirring constantly. When apples are light brown in color, add raisins and keep stirring for about one minute. Add artificial sweetener and sprinkle with a pinch of cinnamon. Mix thoroughly and serve.

Makes one or two servings. Entire recipe contains the following:
Calories: 411   Carbs(g): 60   Protein(g): 9   Fat(g): 21

MEGA-VITAMIN, LOW-CALORIE, NO-FAT SOUP
CLARE FURR (U.S. AND WORLD CHAMPION, FIFTH-PLACE FINISHER, MS. OLYMPIA)

Ingredients:
1 29-ounce can tomato sauce
2–3 29-ounce cans water (amount depends on desired thickness of soup)
1 12-ounce can tomato paste
10 bouillon cubes
1–2 tablespoons garlic powder
2–3 tablespoons Italian seasoning

Stir foregoing ingredients together in an 8- or 10-quart pot over a low heat until blended. When blended, add:

1 12-ounce box frozen squash
1 16-ounce box frozen broccoli
1 16-ounce box frozen cut green beans
2 16-ounce bags frozen cauliflower
1 16-ounce bag frozen sliced yellow squash
2 16-ounce bags frozen sliced carrots

Cover and cook on low heat overnight. (When I'm not dieting for a competition, I will add lima beans, pasta, or small potatoes.) Serve sprinkled with garlic and onion croutons.

Makes approximately four 16-ounce servings. Each serving contains the following:
Calories: 275   Carbs(g): 57   Protein(g): 12   Fat(g): —

SEVICHE

CHRIS GLASS (LOS ANGELES CHAMPION, CALIFORNIA LIGHTWEIGHT CHAMPION)

Ingredients:
1½ pounds scallops
¾ cup fresh lemon juice
¾ cup fresh lime juice
1 teaspoon salt (optional)
¼ teaspoon pepper
½ teaspoon oregano
½ teaspoon garlic powder
1 fresh hot chili pepper (seeded and cut into pieces)
1 medium-sized tomato (chopped)
1 bell pepper (chopped)

Cut scallops into small chunks. Place into a mixing bowl. Add lemon and lime juice. Marinate for six hours, or until fish is white in color (like cooked fish). Drain and rinse marinade. Add other ingredients. Let sit for two to three hours in refrigerator. Garnish with salsa. Serve on a bed of shredded lettuce.

Makes one serving. Each serving contains the following:
Calories: 340   Carbs(g): 26   Protein(g): 54   Fat(g): 5

BROILED RED SNAPPER
RUFUS HOWARD (MR. AMERICA)

Ingredients:
1 pound red snapper
juice of ½ lemon
¼ teaspoon garlic powder
¼ teaspoon onion powder
¼ teaspoon paprika
¼ teaspoon pepper

Place fish on broiler pan. Squeeze juice of one-half lemon over it. Add garlic powder, onion powder, paprika, and pepper. Broil for approximately eight minutes. There is no need to turn the fish. Serve with steamed rice.

Makes one serving. With one cup of cooked rice, one serving contains the following:
Calories: 650   Carbs(g): 50   Protein(g): 93   Fat(g): 5

BROILED HALIBUT STEAK

SEAN PAUL JENKINS (U.S. AND WORLD GAMES MIDDLEWEIGHT CHAMPION)

Ingredients:
1 pound halibut
2 slices onion
2 slices bell pepper
cayenne pepper
lemon pepper

Place fish in broiler pan with onion, pepper, and seasonings. Broil for 15 minutes. Serve on top of brown rice with steamed vegetables. Cook one cup of brown rice according to package directions, and steam eight ounces of broccoli.

Makes one serving. With rice and broccoli one serving contains the following:
Calories: 750   Carbs(g): 59   Protein(g): 105   Fat(g): 5

DELIGHTFUL BREAST

MARY ELLEN JERUMBO (NATIONAL MIDDLEWEIGHT CHAMPION)

Ingredients:
1 4-ounce chicken breast (boned and skinned)
1 cup uncooked minute rice
1 medium-sized tomato (chopped)
1 small onion (chopped)
1 teaspoon garlic powder
juice of ½ lemon
liquid lecithin (can be found in most health food stores)

Pour minute rice in the bottom of a 4 × 4-inch pan lined with liquid lecithin. Place chicken breast in the middle of pan. In separate bowl mix together chopped tomato, onion, and garlic powder. Add lemon juice and mix thoroughly. Pour this mixture over chicken breast and rice. Place in an oven preheated at 350 degrees for approximately 45 minutes, or until the chicken breast is brown. (For the first 20 minutes cover with foil, then remove the foil to brown the chicken.)

Makes one serving. Each serving contains the following:
Calories: 200   Carbs(g): 17   Protein(g): 20   Fat(g): 4

STUFFED BAKED POTATO

KEVIN LAWRENCE (NATIONAL, AMERICAN, AND WORLD MIXED PAIRS CHAMPION)

Ingredients:
2 large potatoes
4 ounces broccoli
½ pound chicken breast

Wash and dry potatoes. Wrap in foil. Place in preheated oven at 350 degrees for 50–60 minutes. While potatoes are baking, steam broccoli in ½ cup water, drain and cut into bite-sized pieces. Broil skinned chicken breast for four minutes on each side, and cut it into bite-sized pieces. When potatoes are done, slice tops open and spoon out potato into medium-sized mixing bowl, leaving foil and skin intact as a shell. Add broccoli and chicken to potato and mix thoroughly. Place mixture back into potato skin and reheat for about five minutes.

Makes two servings Each serving contains the following:
Calories: 355   Carbs(g): 34   Protein(g): 42   Fat(g): 9

CALAMARI STEAKS

GARY LEONARD (MR. AMERICA)

Ingredients:
4 ½-pound calamari (squid) steaks
½ cup seasoned bread crumbs
1 egg lightly beaten
oil or Pam
pesto, made as follows:
   2 bunches fresh basil
   5 cloves garlic
   3 ounces freshly grated Parmesan cheese
   salt to taste
   ½ teaspoon pepper

In food processor or blender finely chop clean basil tops. Add garlic, pepper, and salt. Blend. Add cheese, and mix into basil mixture. Divide pesto mixture evenly. Place one-fourth of mixture on each steak and smooth over. Roll up. Dip in egg, roll in bread crumbs. Place in hot oil or Pam. Brown lightly, turning constantly. After browning, place in baking dish. Bake for 15 minutes at 350 degrees. Can be served with rice or baked potato.

Makes two servings. Each serving contains the following:
Calories: 440   Carbs(g): 31   Protein(g): 48   Fat(g): 10

FRIJOLES

SUE ANN McKEAN (CALIFORNIA CHAMPION)

Ingredients:
2 cups pinto beans
1 pound ground beef
2 medium-sized onions (chopped)
1 stalk celery (chopped)
1 green bell pepper (chopped)
1 1arge clove garlic (chopped)
2 cans tomato sauce
1 bay leaf
salt and pepper to taste
Tabasco to taste
Oregano to taste

Rinse beans before use. Soak two cups pinto beans in six cups of water overnight. Salt water and simmer in same water until beans are barely tender. Taste and add more salt if necessary, but the beans should be bland. Brown meat in a frying pan, add onion, garlic, celery, and green bell pepper. Cook until onion is clear. Pour off fat. Drain off some bean water until the top layer of beans is exposed. Add two cans of tomato sauce, sautéed vegetables, and meat. Add bay leaf, salt and pepper and simmer for one hour. Add Tabasco and oregano to taste after beans have been cooked for one hour.

Makes four large servings. Each serving contains the following:
Calories: 585   Carbs(g): 71   Protein(g): 46   Fat(g): 12

DONNA'S LOW-CAL FISH ROLL-UPS

DONA OLIVEIRA (U.S. AND WORLD GAMES CHAMPION)

Ingredients:
6 4-ounce fillets of sole or flounder
Stuffing for fish
¾ cup scallops (or shrimp, lobster, crab)
⅓ cup Imperial Light Spread
1 cup bread crumbs
1 small onion
1 tablespoon parsley
Additional ingredients
¼ teaspoon pepper
½ teaspoon thyme
¼ teaspoon garlic powder
¼ teaspoon coriander or mace
¼ teaspoon paprika (or amount to taste)
lemon juice

Sauté onion and finely chopped scallops in margarine. Add seasoning and cook for one minute. Mix in bread crumbs. Spread evenly on each fillet, add a few drops of lemon juice over dressing. Roll each fillet jelly-roll fashion. Skewer with toothpicks. Dot each roll with one teaspoon margarine. Place on a cookie sheet and bake in a preheated oven at 350 degrees for 10–15 minutes, or until fish flakes easily when touched with a fork.

Makes two servings. Each serving contains the following:
Calories: 300   Carbs(g): 43   Proteins(g): 24   Fat(g): 10

MARSHA'S MOUTH-WATERING SALAD

MARSHA RADFORD (AMERICAN LIGHTWEIGHT CHAMPION)

Ingredients:
½ cup unsweetened orange juice
2 tablespoons lemon juice
3 individual packets of artificial sweetener
1 medium red apple (diced with peeling)
1 medium green or yellow apple (diced with peeling)
1 cup white seedless grapes or 4 cups raisins
1 banana (sliced)
1 16-ounce can unsweetened pineapple chunks (drained)
1 peach (in season—diced)

Mix orange juice, lemon juice, and artificial sweetener in mixing bowl. Mix all fruit except banana and raisins together. Add liquid and mix well. Refrigerate several hours or overnight. Add sliced banana and raisins 50 minutes before serving. Garnish with strawberry or parsley. (For holidays and special events, add ½ cup chopped pecans and four sliced maraschino cherries.)

Makes six servings. Each serving contains the following:
Calories: 600   Carbs(g): 150   Protein(g): 3   Fat(g): 2

THREE-FRUIT FISH SALAD

JULIE STANGL (MINNESOTA CHAMPION)

Ingredients:
½ large pineapple
1 can mandarin oranges
12 green seedless grapes (halved)
10 large purple grapes (halved)
10 large red grapes (halved)
salad greens
¼ cup slivered almonds
1½ cups cooked halibut, shrimp, crab, or tuna

Cut pineapple in small cubes and place in large bowl with some juice. Add oranges, grapes, and fish. Toss with salad greens and sprinkle top with almonds.

Makes four servings. One serving (using halibut) contains the following:
Calories: 285   Carbs(g): 35   Protein(g): 26   Fat(g): 6

HIGH-PROTEIN, NO-FAT BEANS AND RICE
STEVE TIMMRECK (LOUISIANA AND GREATER GULF STATES CHAMPION)

Ingredients:
1 1-pound bag dried beans (lima, white, red, or black beans—recipe is using lima beans)
10 bouillon cubes
1 medium-sized onion
1 teaspoon garlic powder
¼ cup parsley flakes
1 tablespoon Worcestershire sauce (optional)
8–10 cups water

Soak beans in 8–10 cups water for one to two hours. Drain. In a large pot, add 8–10 cups water, 10 bouillon cubes, onion, garlic powder, parsley flakes, Worcestershire sauce. Cover and cook over low heat for five to six hours.

For rice:
    1 cup white rice
    2 cups water

Bring water to a boil over high heat. Turn heat to low and add rice. Cover and simmer for about 20 minutes. Serve beans over rice.

Makes two servings. Each serving contains the following:
Calories: 415   Carbs(g): 81   Protein(g): 18   Fat(g): 1

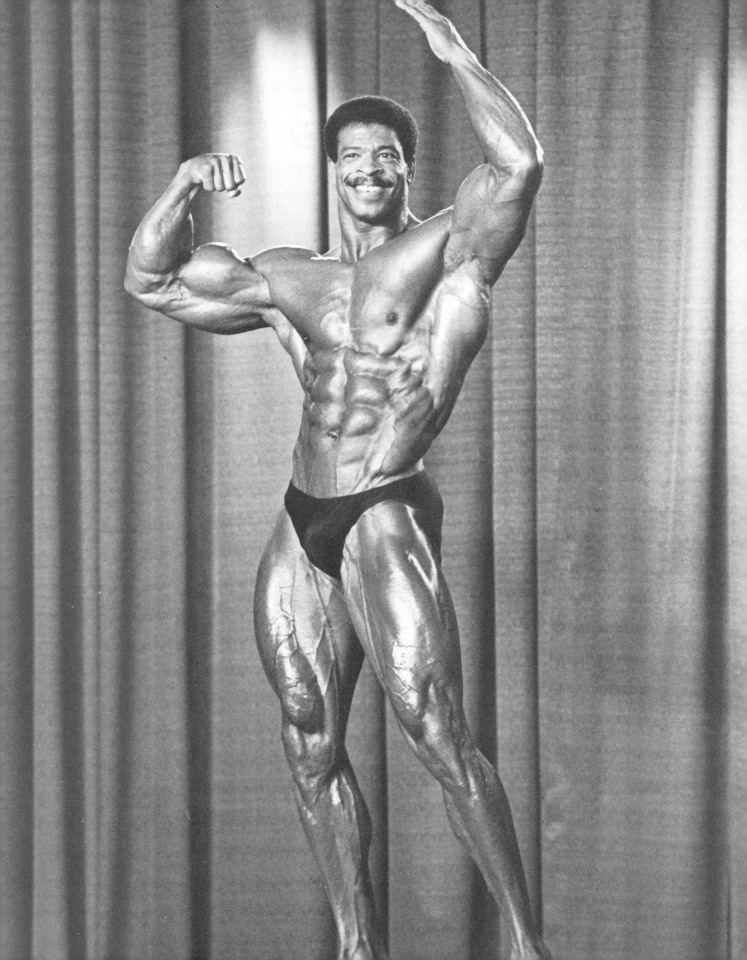

SUGGESTED READINGS

Bannout, Samir, with Bill Reynolds. *Mr. Olympia's Muscle Mastery*. New York: New American Library, 1985.

Brody, Jane. *Jane Brody's Nutrition Book*. New York: Bantam Books, 1982.

Columbu, Dr. Franco, with Lydia Fragomeni. *The Bodybuilder's Nutrition Book*. Chicago: Contemporary Books, 1985.

Darden, Ellington. *The Nautilus Nutrition Book*. Chicago: Contemporary Books, 1981.

Grymkowski, Peter, Edward Connors, Tim Kimber, and Bill Reynolds. *The Gold's Gym Training Encyclopedia*. Chicago: Contemporary Books, 1984.

Kennedy, Robert, and Dennis C. Weis. *Mass! New Scientific Bodybuilding Secrets*. Chicago: Contemporary Books, 1986.

McLish, Rachel, with Bill Reynolds. *Flex Appeal by Rachel*. New York: Warner Books, 1984.

Platz, Tom, with Bill Reynolds. *Pro-Style Bodybuilding*. New York: Sterling Publishing, 1985.

Reynolds, Bill, Peter Grymkowski, Edward Connors, and Tim Kimber. *Solid Gold: Training the Gold's Gym Way*. Chicago: Contemporary Books, 1985.

Reynolds, Bill, and Joyce L. Vedral. *Supercut: Nutrition for the Ultimate Physique*. Chicago: Contemporary Books, 1985.

Schwarzenegger, Arnold, with Bill Dobbins. *Encyclopedia of Modern Bodybuilding*. New York: Simon and Schuster, 1985.

Sprague, Ken, and Bill Reynolds. *The Gold's Gym Book of Bodybuilding*. Chicago: Contemporary Books, 1983.

Walczak, Michael, and Benjamin B. Ehrich. *Nutrition and Well-Being*. Reseda, Calif.: Mojave Books, 1976.

Weider, Joe, ed. *Bodybuilding Nutrition and Training Programs*. Chicago: Contemporary Books, 1981.

————. *More Bodybuilding Nutrition and Training Programs*. Chicago: Contemporary Books, 1982.

Zale, Norman. *Eating for Strength and Development*. Alliance, Nebr.: Iron Man Industries, 1977.

Zane, Frank, and Christina Zane. *Zane Nutrition*. New York: Simon and Schuster, 1986.

INDEX